Integrated Management of Pregnancy and Childbirth

Pregnancy, Childbirth, Postpartum and Newborn Care: A guide for essential practice

Third Edition

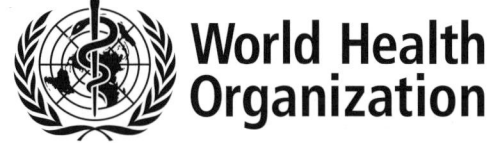

WHO Library Cataloguing-in-Publication Data

Pregnancy, childbirth, postpartum and newborn care: a guide for essential practice – 3rd ed.

    1.Labor, Obstetric. 2.Delivery, Obstetric. 3.Prenatal Care. 4.Perinatal Care. 5.Postnatal Care. 6.Pregnancy Complications. 7.Practice Guideline. I.World Health Organization. II.UNFPA. III.UNICEF. IV.World Bank.

    ISBN 978 92 4 154935 6   (NLM classification: WQ 176)

© World Health Organization 2015

All rights reserved. Publications of the World Health Organization are available on the WHO website (www.who.int) or can be purchased from WHO Press, World Health Organization, 20 Avenue Appia, 1211 Geneva 27, Switzerland (tel.: +41 22 791 3264; fax: +41 22 791 4857; e-mail: bookorders@who.int).

Requests for permission to reproduce or translate WHO publications –whether for sale or for non-commercial distribution– should be addressed to WHO Press through the WHO website (www.who.int/about/licensing/copyright_form/en/index.html).

The designations employed and the presentation of the material in this publication do not imply the expression of any opinion whatsoever on the part of the World Health Organization concerning the legal status of any country, territory, city or area or of its authorities, or concerning the delimitation of its frontiers or boundaries. Dotted and dashed lines on maps represent approximate border lines for which there may not yet be full agreement.

The mention of specific companies or of certain manufacturers' products does not imply that they are endorsed or recommended by the World Health Organization in preference to others of a similar nature that are not mentioned. Errors and omissions excepted, the names of proprietary products are distinguished by initial capital letters.

All reasonable precautions have been taken by the World Health Organization to verify the information contained in this publication. However, the published material is being distributed without warranty of any kind, either expressed or implied. The responsibility for the interpretation and use of the material lies with the reader. In no event shall the World Health Organization be liable for damages arising from its use.

Printed in Luxembourg.

PREFACE

'Pregnancy, Childbirth, Postpartum and Newborn Care: A guide for essential practice' (PCPNC) has been updated to include recommendations from recently approved WHO guidelines relevant to maternal and perinatal health. These include pre-eclampsia & eclampsia; postpartum haemorrhage; postnatal care for the mother and baby; newborn resuscitation; prevention of mother-to- child transmission of HIV; HIV and infant feeding; malaria in pregnancy, tobacco use and second-hand exposure in pregnancy, post-partum depression, post-partum family planning and post abortion care.

This revised guide brings a full range of updated evidence – based norms and standards that enable health care providers at the first health care level to provide high-quality, integrated care during pregnancy and childbirth and after birth, both for mothers and babies. This guide will support countries in their efforts to reach every woman and child and ensure that pregnancy, birth and the first postnatal weeks are the joyful and safe experience they should be. The guide will be updated periodically as new WHO recommendations become available.

This guide represents a common understanding between WHO, UNFPA, UNICEF, and the World Bank of key elements of an approach to reducing maternal and perinatal mortality and morbidity. These agencies co-operate closely in efforts to reduce maternal and perinatal mortality and morbidity. The principles and policies of each agency are governed by the relevant decisions of each agency's governing body and each agency implements the interventions described in this document in accordance with these principles and policies and within the scope of its mandate.

Acknowledgements

ACKNOWLEDGEMENTS

The 2006 edition was prepared by a team of the World Health Organization, Department of Reproductive Health and Research (RHR), led by Jerker Liljestrand and Jelka Zupan.
The concept and first drafts were developed by Sandra Gove and Patricia Whitesell/ACT International, Atlanta, Jerker Liljestrand, Denise Roth, Betty Sweet, Anne Thompson, and Jelka Zupan.
Revisions were subsequently carried out by Annie Portela, Luc de Bernis, Ornella Lincetto, Rita Kabra, Maggie Usher, Agostino Borra, Rick Guidotti, Elisabeth Hoff, Mathews Matthai, Monir Islam, Felicity Savage, Adepeyu Olukoya, Aafje Rietveld, TinTin Sint, Ekpini Ehounou, Suman Mehta.

Valuable inputs were provided by WHO Regional Offices and WHO departments:

- Reproductive Health and Research (RHR)
- Maternal, Newborn, Child and Adolescent Health (MCA)
- HIV/AIDS
- Nutrition for Health and Development (NHD)
- Essential Medicines and Health Products (EMP)
- Immunization, Vaccines and Biologicals (IVB)
- Mental Health and Substance Abuse (MSD)
- Gender, Women and Health (GWH)
- Prevention of Blindness and Deafness (PBD)
- Prevention of Noncommunicable Diseases (PND)

Editing: Nina Mattock, Richard Casna
Layout: rsdesigns.com sàrl
Cover design: Maíre Ní Mhearáin

WHO acknowledges with gratitude the generous contribution of over 100 individuals and organizations in the field of maternal and newborn health, who took time to review the 2006 version at different stages of its development. They came from over 35 countries and brought their expertise and wide experience to the final text.

The guide was also reviewed and endorsed by the International Confederation of Midwives, the International Federation of Gynecology and Obstetrics and International Pediatric Association.

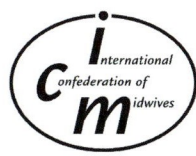
International Confederation of Midwives

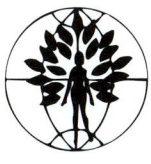
International Federation of Gynecology and Obstetrics

International Pediatric Association

The financial support towards the preparation and production of the 2006 version was provided by UNFPA, the World Bank and the Governments of Australia, Japan and the United States of America.

The present version was revised and updated by Jelka Zupan and Juana Willumsen. Overall technical direction and supervision of the document was maintained by Maurice Bucagu of WHO/MCA.

Technical inputs were provided by Matthews Mathai, Annie portela, severin von Xylander, Metin Ahmet Gulmezoglu, Bela Ganatra, Mercedes Semenas Bonet, Taiwo Olufemi Oladapo, Ehizibue Peter Olumese, Susheela Engelbrecht, Fabio Uxa, Patricia Coffey, Satvinder Singh, Mustafa Shaffiq Essajee, Ahmadu Yakubu. Financial support for the update was provided by The Norwegian Agency for Development Cooperation and Ministry of Foreign Affairs and International Development (France).

TABLE OF CONTENTS

INTRODUCTION

- **i** Introduction
- **i2** How to read the Guide
- **i3** Structure and presentation
- **i4** Assumptions underlying the guide

A PRINCIPLES OF GOOD CARE

- **A2** Communication
- **A3** Workplace and administrative procedures
- **A4** Standard precautions and cleanliness
- **A5** Organising a visit

B QUICK CHECK, RAPID ASSESSMENT AND MANAGEMENT OF WOMEN OF CHILDBEARING AGE

- **B2** Quick check
- **B3-B7** Rapid assessment and management
  - **B3** Airway and breathing
  - **B3** Circulation (shock)
  - **B4-B5** Vaginal bleeding
  - **B6** Convulsions or unconscious
  - **B6** Severe abdominal pain
  - **B6** Dangerous fever
  - **B7** Labour
  - **B7** Other danger signs or symptoms
  - **B7** If no emergency or priority signs, non urgent

B EMERGENCY TREATMENTS FOR THE WOMAN

- **B9** Airway, breathing and circulation
  - **B9** Manage the airway and breathing
  - **B9** Insert IV line and give fluids
  - **B9** If intravenous access not possible
- **B10-B12** Bleeding
  - **B10** Massage uterus and expel clots
  - **B10** Apply bimanual uterine compression
  - **B10** Apply aortic compression
  - **B10** Give oxytocin
  - **B10** Give misoprostol
  - **B10** Give ergometrine
  - **B11** Remove placenta and fragments manually
  - **B11** After manual removal of placenta
  - **B12** Repair the tear or episiotomy
  - **B12** Empty bladder
- **B13-B14** Important considerations in caring for a woman with eclampsia or pre-eclampsia
  - **B13** Give magnesium sulphate
  - **B13** Important considerations in caring for a woman with eclampsia
  - **B14** Give diazepam
  - **B14** Give appropriate antihypertensive drug
- **B15** Infection
  - **B15** Give appropriate IV/IM antibiotics
- **B16** Malaria
  - **B16** Treatment of uncomplicated P.falciparum malaria in pregnancy
- **B17** Refer the woman urgently to the hospital
  - **B17** Essential emergency drugs and supplies for transport and home delivery

B BLEEDING IN EARLY PREGNANCY AND POST-ABORTION CARE

- **B19** Examination of the woman with bleeding in early pregnancy and post-abortion care
- **B20** Give preventive measures
- **B21** Advise and counsel on post-abortion care
  - **B21** Advise on self-care
  - **B21** Advise and counsel on family planning
  - **B21** Provide information and support after abortion
  - **B21** Advise and counsel during follow-up visits

Table of contents

C ANTENATAL CARE

- **C2** Assess the pregnant woman: pregnancy status, birth and emergency plan
  - **C3** Check for pre-eclampsia
  - **C4** Check for anaemia
  - **C5** Check for syphilis
  - **C6** Check for HIV status
- **C7** Respond to observed signs or volunteered problems
  - **C7** If no fetal movement
  - **C7** If ruptured membranes and no labour
  - **C8** If fever or burning on urination
  - **C9** If vaginal discharge
  - **C10** If signs suggesting HIV infection
  - **C10** If smoking, alcohol or drug abuse, or history of violence
  - **C11** If cough or breathing difficulty
  - **C11** If taking antituberculosis drugs
- **C12** Give preventive measures
- **C13** Advise and counsel on nutrition and self-care
- **C14-C15** Develop a birth and emergency plan
  - **C14** Facility delivery
  - **C14** Home delivery with a skilled attendant
  - **C15** Advise on labour signs
  - **C15** Advise on danger signs
  - **C15** Discuss how to prepare for an emergency in pregnancy
- **C16** Advise and counsel on family planning
  - **C16** Counsel on the importance of family planning
  - **C16** Special consideration for family planning counselling during pregnancy
- **C17** Advise on routine and follow-up visits
- **C18** Home delivery without a skilled attendant

D CHILDBIRTH – LABOUR, DELIVERY AND IMMEDIATE POSTPARTUM CARE

- **D2** Examine the woman in labour or with ruptured membranes
- **D3** Decide stage of labour
- **D4-D5** Respond to obstetrical problems on admission
- **D6-D7** Give supportive care throughout labour
  - **D6** Communication
  - **D6** Cleanliness
  - **D6** Mobility
  - **D6** Urination
  - **D6** Eating, drinking
  - **D6** Breathing technique
  - **D6** Pain and discomfort relief
  - **D7** Birth companion
- **D8-D9** First stage of labour
  - **D8** Not in active labour
  - **D9** In active labour
- **D10-D11** Second stage of labour: deliver the baby and give immediate newborn care
- **D12-D13** Third stage of labour: deliver the placenta
- **D14-D18** Respond to problems during labour and delivery
  - **D14** If fetal heart rate <120 or >160 beats per minute
  - **D15** If prolapsed cord
  - **D16** If breech presentation
  - **D17** If stuck shoulders (Shoulder dystocia)
  - **D18** If multiple births
- **D19** Care of the mother and newborn within first hour of delivery of placenta
- **D20** Care of the mother one hour after delivery of placenta
- **D21** Assess the mother after delivery
- **D22-D25** Respond to problems immediately postpartum
  - **D22** If vaginal bleeding
  - **D22** If fever (temperature >38°C)
  - **D22** If perineal tear or episiotomy (done for lifesaving circumstances)
  - **D23** If elevated diastolic blood pressure
  - **D24** If pallor on screening, check for anaemia
  - **D24** If mother severely ill or separated from the child
  - **D24** If baby stillborn or dead
- **D25** Give preventive measures

D CHILDBIRTH – LABOUR, DELIVERY AND IMMEDIATE POSTPARTUM CARE (CONTINUED)

- **D26** Advise on postpartum care
  - **D26** Advise on postpartum care and hygiene
  - **D26** Counsel on nutrition
- **D27** Counsel on birth spacing and family planning
  - **D27** Counsel on the importance of family planning
  - **D27** Lactation amenorrhea method (LAM)
- **D28** Advise on when to return
  - **D28** Routine postpartum visits
  - **D28** Follow-up visits for problems
  - **D28** Advise on danger signs
  - **D28** Discuss how to prepare for an emergency in postpartum
- **D29** Home delivery by skilled attendant
  - **D29** Preparation for home delivery
  - **D29** Delivery care
  - **D29** Immediate postpartum care of mother
  - **D29** Postpartum care of newborn

E POSTPARTUM CARE

- **E2** Postpartum examination of the mother (up to 6 weeks)
- **E3-E10** Respond to observed signs or volunteered problems
  - **E3** If elevated diastolic blood pressure
  - **E4** If pallor, check for anaemia
  - **E5** Check for HIV status
  - **E6** If heavy vaginal bleeding
  - **E6** If fever or foul-smelling lochia
  - **E7** If dribbling urine
  - **E7** If pus or perineal pain
  - **E7** If feeling unhappy or crying easily
  - **E8** If vaginal discharge 4 weeks after delivery
  - **E8** If breast problem
  - **E9** If cough or breathing difficulty
  - **E9** If taking anti-tuberculosis drugs
  - **E10** If signs suggesting HIV infection

F PREVENTIVE MEASURES AND ADDITIONAL TREATMENTS FOR THE WOMAN

- **F2–F4** Preventive measures
  - **F2** Give tetanus toxoid
  - **F2** Give iron and folic acid
  - **F2** Give mebendazole
  - **F3** Give aspirin and calcium (if in area of low dietary calcium intake)
  - **F3** Motivate on adherence with treatments
  - **F4** Give preventive intermittent treatment for falciparum malaria in pregnancy
  - **F4** Advise to use insecticide-treated bednet
  - **F4** Give appropriate oral antimalarial treatment (uncomplicated P. falciparum malaria)
  - **F4** Give paracetamol
- **F5–F6** Additional treatments for the woman
  - **F5** Give appropriate oral antibiotics
  - **F6** Give benzathine penicillin IM
  - **F6** Observe for signs of allergy

Table of contents

Table of contents

G — INFORM AND COUNSEL ON HIV

- **G2** Provide key information on HIV
  - **G2** What is HIV and how is HIV transmitted?
  - **G2** Advantage of knowing the HIV status in pregnancy
  - **G2** Counsel on safer sex including use of condoms
- **G3** HIV testing and counselling
  - **G3** HIV testing and counselling
  - **G3** Discuss confidentiality of HIV infection
  - **G3** Counsel on implications of the HIV test result
  - **G3** Benefits of disclosure (involving) and testing the male partner(s)
- **G4** Care and counselling for the HIV-infected woman
  - **G4** Additional care for the HIV-infected woman
  - **G4** Counsel the HIV-infected woman on family planning
- **G5** Support to the HIV-infected woman
  - **G5** Provide emotional support to the woman
  - **G5** How to provide support
- **G6** Give antiretroviral medicine (ART) to treat HIV infection
  - **G6** Support the initiation of ART
  - **G6** Support adherence to ART
- **G7** Counsel on infant feeding options
  - **G7** Explain the risks of HIV transmission through breastfeeding and not breastfeeding
  - **G7** If a woman does not know her HIV status
  - **G7** If a woman knows that she is HIV infected
  - **G7** Give special counselling to the mother who is HIV-infected and chooses breastfeeding
- **G8** Support the mothers choice of newborn feeding
  - **G8** If mother chooses replacement feeding : teach her replacement feeding
  - **G8** Explain the risks of replacement feeding
  - **G8** Follow-up for replacement feeding
- **G9** Antiretroviral medicines (ART) to HIV-infected woman and the newborn
- **G10** Respond to observed signs and volunteered problems
  - **G10** If a woman is taking Antiretroviral medicines and develop new signs/symptoms, respond to her problems
- **G11** Prevent HIV infection in health care workers after accidental exposure with body fluids (post exposure prophylaxis)
  - **G11** If a health care worker is exposed to body fluids by cuts/pricks/ splashes, give him appropriate care.
- **G12** Give antiretroviral medicines (ART) to the HIV-infected woman and her baby

H — THE WOMAN WITH SPECIAL NEEDS

- **H2** Emotional support for the woman with special needs
  - **H2** Sources of support
  - **H2** Emotional support
- **H3** Special considerations in managing the pregnant adolescent
  - **H3** When interacting with the adolescent
  - **H3** Help the girl consider her options and to make decisions which best suit her needs
- **H4** Special considerations for supporting the woman living with violence
  - **H4** Support the woman living with violence
  - **H4** Support the health service response to needs of women living with violence

I — COMMUNITY SUPPORT FOR MATERNAL AND NEWBORN HEALTH

- **I2** Establish links
  - **I2** Coordinate with other health care providers and community groups
  - **I2** Establish links with traditional birth attendants and traditional healers
- **I3** Involve the community in quality of services

J NEWBORN CARE

- **J2** Examine the newborn
  - **J3** If preterm, birth weight <2500 g or twin
  - **J4** Assess breastfeeding
  - **J5** Check for special treatment needs
  - **J6** Look for signs of jaundice and local infection
  - **J7** If danger signs
  - **J8** If swelling, bruises or malformation
  - **J9** Assess the mother's breasts if complaining of nipple or breast pain
- **J10** Care of the newborn
- **J11** Additional care of a small baby (or twin)
- **J12** Assess replacement feeding

K BREASTFEEDING, CARE, PREVENTIVE MEASURES AND TREATMENT FOR THE NEWBORN

- **K2** Counsel on breastfeeding
  - **K2** Counsel on importance of exclusive breastfeeding
  - **K2** Help the mother to initiate breastfeeding
  - **K3** Support exclusive breastfeeding
  - **K3** Teach correct positioning and attachment for breastfeeding
  - **K4** Give special support to breastfeed the small baby (preterm and/or low birth weight)
  - **K4** Give special support to breastfeed twins
- **K5** Alternative feeding methods
  - **K5** Express breast milk
  - **K5** Hand express breast milk directly into the baby's mouth
  - **K6** Cup feeding expressed breast milk
  - **K6** Teach mother heat treating expressed breast milk
  - **K6** Quantity to feed by cup
  - **K6** Signs that baby is receiving adequate amount of milk
- **K7** Weigh and assess weight gain
  - **K7** Weigh baby in the first month of life
  - **K7** Assess weight gain
  - **K7** Scale maintenance
- **K8** Other breastfeeding support
  - **K8** Give special support to the mother who is not yet breastfeeding
  - **K8** If the baby does not have a mother
  - **K8** Advise the mother who is not breastfeeding at all on how to relieve engorgement
- **K9** Ensure warmth for the baby
  - **K9** Keep the baby warm
  - **K9** Keep a small baby warm
  - **K9** Rewarm the baby skin-to-skin
- **K10** Other baby care
  - **K10** Cord care
  - **K10** Sleeping
  - **K10** Hygiene
- **K11** Newborn resuscitation
  - **K11** Keep the baby warm
  - **K11** Open the airway
  - **K11** If still not breathing, ventilate
  - **K11** If breathing less than 30 breaths per minute or severe chest in-drawing, stop ventilating
  - **K11** If not breathing or gasping at all after 20 minutes of ventilation
- **K12** Treat and immunize the baby
  - **K12** Treat the baby
  - **K12** Give 2 IM antibiotics (first week of life)
  - **K12** Give IM benzathine penicillin to baby (single dose) if mother tested RPR-positive
  - **K12** Give IM antibiotic for possible gonococcal eye infection (single dose)
  - **K13** Teach the mother to give treatment to the baby at home
  - **K13** Treat local infection
  - **K13** Give isoniazid (INH) prophylaxis to newborn
  - **K13** Immunize the newborn
  - **K13** Give antiretroviral (ARV) medicine to newborn
- **K14** Advise when to return with the baby
  - **K14** Routine visits
  - **K14** Follow-up visits
  - **K14** Advise the mother to seek care for the baby
  - **K14** Refer baby urgently to hospital

Table of contents

Table of contents

L EQUIPMENT, SUPPLIES, DRUGS AND LABORATORY TESTS

- **L2** Equipment, supplies, drugs and tests for pregnancy and postpartum care
- **L3** Equipment, supplies and drugs for childbirth care
- **L4** Laboratory tests
  - **L4** Check urine for protein
  - **L4** Check haemoglobin
- **L5** Perform rapid plamareagin (RPR) test for syphilis
  - **L5** Interpreting results
- **L6** Perform rapid test for HIV

M INFORMATION AND COUNSELLING SHEETS

- **M2** Care during pregnancy
- **M3** Preparing a birth and emergency plan
- **M4** Care for the mother after birth
- **M5** Care after an abortion
- **M6** Care for the baby after birth
- **M7** Breastfeeding
- **M8-M9** Clean home delivery

N RECORDS AND FORMS

- **N2** Referral record
- **N3** Feedback record
- **N4** Labour record
- **N5** Partograph
- **N6** Postpartum record
- **N7** International form of medical certificate of cause of death

GLOSSARY AND ACRONYMS

INTRODUCTION

The aim of Pregnancy, childbirth, postpartum and newborn care guide for essential practice (PCPNC) is to provide evidence-based recommendations to guide health care professionals in the management of women during pregnancy, childbirth and postpartum, and post abortion, and newborns during their first week of life, including management of endemic diseases like malaria, HIV/AIDS, TB and anaemia.

All recommendations are for skilled attendants working at the primary level of health care, either at the facility or in the community. They apply to all women attending antenatal care, in delivery, postpartum or post abortion care, or who come for emergency care, and to all newborns at birth and during the first week of life (or later) for routine and emergency care.

The PCPNC is a guide for clinical decision-making. It facilitates the collection, analysis, classification and use of relevant information by suggesting key questions, essential observations and/or examinations, and recommending appropriate research-based interventions. It promotes the early detection of complications and the initiation of early and appropriate treatment, including timely referral, if necessary.

Correct use of this guide should help reduce the high maternal and perinatal mortality and morbidity rates prevalent in many parts of the developing world, thereby making pregnancy and childbirth safer.

The guide is not designed for immediate use. It is a generic guide and should first be adapted to local needs and resources. It should cover the most serious endemic conditions that the skilled birth attendant must be able to treat, and be made consistent with national treatment guidelines and other policies. It is accompanied by an adaptation guide to help countries prepare their own national guides and training and other supporting materials.

The first section, How to use the guide, describes how the guide is organized, the overall content and presentation. Each chapter begins with a short description of how to read and use it, to help the reader use the guide correctly.

The Guide has been developed by the Department of Reproductive Health and Research and the Department of Maternal, Newborn, Child and Adolescent Health with contributions from the following WHO programmes:

- HIV/AIDS
- Nutrition for Health and Development (NHD)
- Essential Medicines and Health Products (EMP)
- Immunization, Vaccines and Biologicals (IVB)
- Mental Health and Substance Abuse (MSD)
- Gender, Women and Health (GWH)
- Prevention of Blindness and Deafness (PBD)
- Prevention of Noncommunicable Diseases (PND)

Introduction

How to read the guide

HOW TO READ THE GUIDE

Content

The Guide includes routine and emergency care for women and newborns during pregnancy, labour and delivery, postpartum and post abortion, as well as key preventive measures required to reduce the incidence of endemic and other diseases like malaria, anaemia, HIV/AIDS and TB, which add to maternal and perinatal morbidity and mortality.

Most women and newborns using the services described in the Guide are not ill and/or do not have complications. They are able to wait in line when they come for a scheduled visit. However, the small proportion of women/newborns who are ill, have complications or are in labour, need urgent attention and care.

The clinical content is divided into six sections which are as follows:
- Quick check (triage), emergency management (called Rapid Assessment and Management or RAM) and referral, followed by a chapter on emergency treatments for the woman.
- Post-abortion care.
- Antenatal care.
- Labour and delivery.
- Postpartum care.
- Newborn care.

In each of the six clinical sections listed above there is a series of flow, treatment and information charts which include:
- Guidance on routine care, including monitoring the well-being of the mother and/or baby.
- Early detection and management of complications.
- Preventive measures.
- Advice and counselling.

In addition to the clinical care outlined above, other sections in the guide include:
- Advice on HIV, prevention and treatment.
- Support for women with special needs.
- Links with the community.
- Drugs, supplies, equipment, universal precautions and laboratory tests.
- Counselling and key messages for women and families.

There is an important section at the beginning of the Guide entitled Principles of good care **A1-A5**. This includes principles of good care for all women, including those with special needs. It explains the organization of each visit to a healthcare facility, which applies to overall care. The principles are not repeated for each visit.

Recommendations for the management of complications at secondary (referral) health care level can be found in the following guides for midwives and doctors:

- Managing complications of pregnancy and childbirth (WHO/RHR/00.7)
- Managing newborn problems.

Documents referred to in this Guide can be obtained from the Department of Maternal, Newborn, Child and Adolescent Health,
World Health Organization, Geneva, Switzerland.
E-mail: mncah@who.int.

Other related WHO documents can be downloaded from the following links:
- World Health Organization. Medical eligibility criteria for contraceptive use. Fifth edition, 2015. http://www.who.int/reproductivehealth/publications/family_planning/MEC-5/en/
- Guidelines for the Management of Sexually Transmitted Infections: http://www.who.int/reproductive-health/publications/rhr_01_10_mngt_stis/guidelines_mngt_stis.pdf
- Sexually Transmitted and other Reproductive Tract Infections: A Guide to Essential Practice: http://www.who.int/reproductive-health/publications/rtis_gep/rtis_gep.pdf
- Consolidated guidelines on the use of antiretroviral drugs for treating and preventing HIV infection. Recommendations for a public health approach. World Health Organization June 2013: http://www.who.int/hiv/pub/guidelines/arv2013/download/en/index.html
- Service delivery approaches to HIV testing and counselling (HTC): a strategic HTC programme framework. World Health Organization 2012. http://www.who.int/
- Malaria and HIV Interactions and their Implications for Public Health Policy. http://www.who.int/hiv/pub/prev_care/en: ISNB 92 4 159335 0
- Interim WHO clinical staging of HIV/AIDS and HIV/AIDS case definitions for surveillance African Region. http://www.who.int/hiv/pub/prev_care/en Ref no: WHO/HIV/2005.02
- HIV and Infant Feeding. Guidelines on HIV and Infant feeding. http://www.who.int/maternal_child_adolescent/documents/9789241599535/en/
- Integrated Management of Adolescent and adult illness http://www.who.int/3by5/publications/documents/imai/en/index.html
- Counselling for maternal and newborn health care: a handbook for building skills. http://www.who.int/maternal_child_adolescent/documents/9789241547628/en/index.html
- Updated WHO policy recommendation: intermittent preventive treatment of malaria in pregnancy using sulfadoxine-pyrimethamine (IPTp-SP). October 2012 http://www.who.int/malaria/publications/atoz/who_iptp_sp_policy_recommendation/en/
- Guidelines for the treatment of malaria. Third edition. April 2015 http://www.who.int/malaria/publications/atoz/9789241547925/en/
- WHO recommendations for the prevention and treatment of postpartum haemorrhage. 2012 http://www.who.int/reproductivehealth/publications/maternal_perinatal_health/9789241548502/en/
- WHO recommendations for prevention and treatment of pre-eclampsia and eclampsia. 2011. http://www.who.int/reproductivehealth/publications/maternal_perinatal_health/9789241548335/en/
- WHO recommendations for the prevention and management of tobacco use and second-hand smoke exposure in pregnancy. http://www.who.int/tobacco/publications/pregnancy/guidelinestobaccosmokeexposure/en/index.html
- Hand hygiene in outpatient and home-based care and long-term care facilities: a guide to the application of the WHO multimodal hand hygiene improvement strategy and the "My Five Moments For Hand Hygiene" approach.
- Vitamin A supplementation in postpartum. Guideline. World Health Organization 2011 http://www.who.int/nutrition/publications/micronutrients/guidelines/vas_postpartum/en/
- WHO recommendations on interventions to improve preterm birth outcomes. World Health Organization 2015. http://apps.who.int/iris/bitstream/10665/183037/1/9789241508988_eng.pdf?ua=1
- WHO guidelines on hand hygiene in healthcare (2009). http://apps.who.int/iris/bitstream/10665/44102/1/9789241597906_eng.pdf.
- WHO recommendations for prevention and treatment of maternal peripartum infections. 2015. http://www.who.int/reproductivehealth/publications/maternal_perinatal_health/peripartum-infections-guidelines/en/.
- 19th WHO Model List of Essential Medicines (April 2015). http://www.who.int/selection_medicines/committees/expert/20/EML_2015_FINAL_amended_AUG2015.pdf?ua=1&ua=1.
- WHO. Safe abortion: technical and policy guidance for health systems. Second edition, 2012. http://www.who.int/reproductivehealth/publications/unsafe_abortion/9789241548434/en/.
- World Health Organization. Consolidated guidelines on the use of antiretroviral drugs for treating and preventing HIV infection: what's new. Policy brief. 2015. http://www.who.int/hiv/pub/arv/policy-brief-arv-
- World Health Organization. WHO recommendations on Postnatal care of the mother and newborn. 2013. http://www.who.int/maternal_child_adolescent/documents/postnatal-care-recommendations/en/
- World Health Organization. Guidelines on basic newborn resuscitation. 2012 http://www.who.int/maternal_child_adolescent/documents/basic_newborn_resuscitation/en/.
- World Health Organization. Pocket book of hospital care for children: Second edition. Guidelines for the management of common childhood illnesses. 2013. http://www.who.int/maternal_child_adolescent/documents/child_hospital_care/en/.

STRUCTURE AND PRESENTATION

This Guide is a tool for clinical decision-making. The content is presented in a frame work of coloured flow charts supported by information and treatment charts which give further details of care.

The framework is based on a syndromic approach whereby the skilled attendant

identifies a limited number of key clinical signs and symptoms, enabling her/him to classify the condition according to severity and give appropriate treatment. Severity is marked in colour: red for emergencies, yellow for less urgent conditions which nevertheless need attention, and green for normal care.

Flow charts

The flow charts include the following information:

1. Key questions to be asked.
2. Important observations and examinations to be made.
3. Possible findings (signs) based on information elicited from the questions, observations and, where appropriate, examinations.
4. Classification of the findings.
5. Treatment and advice related to the signs and classification.

"Treat, advise" means giving the treatment indicated (performing a procedure, prescribing drugs or other treatments, advising on possible side-effects and how to overcome them) and giving advice on other important practices. The treat and advise column is often cross-referenced to other treatment and/or information charts. Turn to these charts for more information.

Use of colour

Colour is used in the flow charts to indicate the severity of a condition.

6. Red highlights an emergency which requires immediate treatment and, in most cases, urgent referral to a higher level health facility.
7. Yellow indicates that there is a problem that can be treated without referral.
8. Green usually indicates no abnormal condition and therefore normal care is given, as outlined in the guide, with appropriate advice for home care and follow up.

Key sequential steps

The charts for normal and abnormal deliveries are presented in a framework of key sequential steps for a clean safe delivery. The key sequential steps for delivery are in a column on the left side of the page, while the column on the right has interventions which may be required if problems arise during delivery. Interventions may be linked to relevant treatment and/or information pages, and are cross-referenced to other parts of the Guide.

Treatment and information pages

The flow charts are linked (cross-referenced) to relevant treatment and/or information pages in other parts of the Guide. These pages include information which is too detailed to include in the flow charts:

- Treatments.
- Advice and counselling.
- Preventive measures.
- Relevant procedures.

Information and counselling sheets

These contain appropriate advice and counselling messages to provide to the woman, her partner and family. In addition, a section is included at the back of the Guide to support the skilled attendant in this effort. Individual sheets are provided with simplified versions of the messages on care during pregnancy (preparing a birth and emergency plan, clean home delivery, care for the mother and baby after delivery, breastfeeding and care after an abortion) to be given to the mother, her partner and family at the appropriate stage of pregnancy and childbirth.

These sheets are presented in a generic format. They will require adaptation to local conditions and language, and the addition of illustrations to enhance understanding, acceptability and attractiveness. Different programmes may prefer a different format such as a booklet or flip chart.

Structure and presentation

Assumptions underlying the Guide

i4

ASSUMPTIONS UNDERLYING THE GUIDE

Recommendations in the Guide are generic, made on many assumptions about the health characteristics of the population and the health care system (the setting, capacity and organization of services, resources and staffing).

Population and endemic conditions

- High maternal and perinatal mortality
- Many adolescent pregnancies
- High prevalence of endemic conditions:
  → Anaemia
  → Stable transmission of falciparum malaria
  → Hookworms (Necator americanus and Ancylostoma duodenale)
  → Sexually transmitted infections, including HIV/AIDS
  → Vitamin A and iron/folate deficiencies

Health care system

The Guide assumes that:
- Routine and emergency pregnancy, delivery and postpartum care are provided at the primary level of the health care, e.g. at the facility near where the woman lives. This facility could be a health post, health centre or maternity clinic. It could also be a hospital with a delivery ward and outpatient clinic providing routine care to women from the neighbourhood.

- A single skilled attendant is providing care. She/he may work at the health care centre, a maternity unit of a hospital or she/he may go to the woman's home, if necessary. However there may be other health workers who receive the woman or support the skilled attendant when emergency complications occur.
- Human resources, infrastructure, equipment, supplies and drugs are limited. However, essential drugs, IV fluids, supplies, gloves and essential equipment are available.
- If a health worker with higher levels of skill (at the facility or a referral hospital) is providing pregnancy, childbirth and postpartum care to women other than those referred, she follows the recommendations described in this Guide.
- Routine visits and follow-up visits are "scheduled" during office hours.
- Emergency services ("unscheduled" visits) for labour and delivery, complications, or severe illness or deterioration are provided 24/24 hours, 7 days a week.
- Women and babies with complications or expected complications are referred for further care to the secondary level of care, a referral hospital.
- Referral and transportation are appropriate for the distance and other circumstances. They must be safe for the mother and the baby.

- Some deliveries are conducted at home, attended by traditional birth attendants (TBAs) or relatives, or the woman delivers alone (but home delivery without a skilled attendant is not recommended).
- Links with the community and traditional providers are established. Primary health care services and the community are involved in maternal and newborn health issues.
- Other programme activities, such as management of malaria, tuberculosis and other lung diseases, treatment for HIV, and infant feeding counselling, that require specific training, are delivered by a different provider, at the same facility or at the referral hospital. Detection, initial treatment and referral are done by the skilled attendant.
- All pregnant woman are routinely offered HIV testing and counselling at the first contact with the health worker, which could be during the antenatal visits, in early labour or in the postpartum period.
  Women who are first seen by the health worker in late labour are offered the test after the childbirth.
  Health workers are trained to provide HIV testing and counselling.
  HIV testing kits and ARV drugs are available at the Primary health-care

Knowledge and skills of care providers

This Guide assumes that professionals using it have the knowledge and skills in providing the care it describes. Other training materials must be used to bring the skills up to the level assumed by the Guide.

Adaptation of the Guide

It is essential that this generic Guide is adapted to not only national and local situations, demographic and epidemiological conditions (e.g. dietary calcium intake among the general population), existing health priorities and resources, but also within the context of respect and sensitivity to the needs of women, newborns and the communities to which they belong.

PRINCIPLES OF GOOD CARE

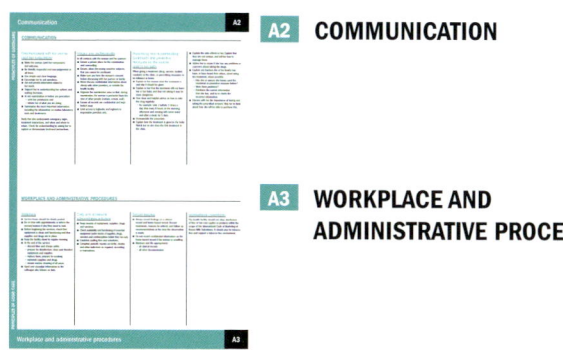

A2 COMMUNICATION

A3 WORKPLACE AND ADMINISTRATIVE PROCEDURES

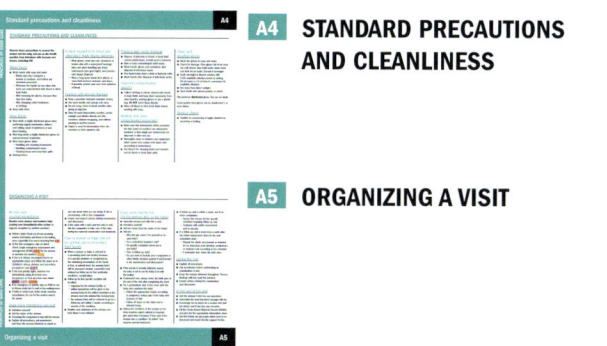

A4 STANDARD PRECAUTIONS AND CLEANLINESS

A5 ORGANIZING A VISIT

These principles of good care apply to all contacts between the skilled attendant and all women and their babies; they are not repeated in each section. Care-givers should therefore familiarize themselves with the following principles before using the Guide. The principles concern:

- Communication **A2**.
- Workplace and administrative procedures **A3**.
- Standard precautions and cleanliness **A4**.
- Organizing a visit **A5**.

Principles of good care

Communication

A2

PRINCIPLES OF GOOD CARE

COMMUNICATION

Communicating with the woman (and her companion)

- Make the woman (and her companion) feel welcome.
- Be friendly, respectful and non-judgmental at all times.
- Use simple and clear language.
- Encourage her to ask questions.
- Ask and provide information related to her needs.
- Support her in understanding her options and making decisions.
- At any examination or before any procedure:
  → seek her permission and
  → inform her of what you are doing.
- Summarize the most important information, including the information on routine laboratory tests and treatments.

Verify that she understands emergency signs, treatment instructions, and when and where to return. Check for understanding by asking her to explain or demonstrate treatment instructions.

Privacy and confidentiality

In all contacts with the woman and her partner:
- Ensure a private place for the examination and counselling.
- Ensure, when discussing sensitive subjects, that you cannot be overheard.
- Make sure you have the woman's consent before discussing with her partner or family.
- Never discuss confidential information about clients with other providers, or outside the health facility.
- Organize the examination area so that, during examination, the woman is protected from the view of other people (curtain, screen, wall).
- Ensure all records are confidential and kept locked away.
- Limit access to logbooks and registers to responsible providers only.

Prescribing and recommending treatments and preventive measures for the woman and/or her baby

When giving a treatment (drug, vaccine, bednet, condom) at the clinic, or prescribing measures to be followed at home:
- Explain to the woman what the treatment is and why it should be given.
- Explain to her that the treatment will not harm her or her baby, and that not taking it may be more dangerous.
- Give clear and helpful advice on how to take the drug regularly:
  → for example: take 2 tablets 3 times a day, thus every 8 hours, in the morning, afternoon and evening with some water and after a meal, for 5 days.
- Demonstrate the procedure.
- Explain how the treatment is given to the baby. Watch her as she does the first treatment in the clinic.
- Explain the side-effects to her. Explain that they are not serious, and tell her how to manage them.
- Advise her to return if she has any problems or concerns about taking the drugs.
- Explore any barriers she or her family may have, or have heard from others, about using the treatment, where possible:
  → Has she or anyone she knows used the treatment or preventive measure before?
  → Were there problems?
  → Reinforce the correct information that she has, and try to clarify the incorrect information.
- Discuss with her the importance of buying and taking the prescribed amount. Help her to think about how she will be able to purchase this.

WORKPLACE AND ADMINISTRATIVE PROCEDURES

Workplace

- Service hours should be clearly posted.
- Be on time with appointments or inform the woman/women if she/they need to wait.
- Before beginning the services, check that equipment is clean and functioning and that supplies and drugs are in place.
- Keep the facility clean by regular cleaning.
- At the end of the service:
  → discard litter and sharps safely
  → prepare for disinfection; clean and disinfect equipment and supplies
  → replace linen, prepare for washing
  → replenish supplies and drugs
  → ensure routine cleaning of all areas.
- Hand over essential information to the colleague who follows on duty.

Daily and occasional administrative activities

- Keep records of equipment, supplies, drugs and vaccines.
- Check availability and functioning of essential equipment (order stocks of supplies, drugs, vaccines and contraceptives before they run out).
- Establish staffing lists and schedules.
- Complete periodic reports on births, deaths and other indicators as required, according to instructions.

Record keeping

- Always record findings on a clinical record and home-based record. Record treatments, reasons for referral, and follow-up recommendations at the time the observation is made.
- Do not record confidential information on the home-based record if the woman is unwilling.
- Maintain and file appropriately:
  → all clinical records
  → all other documentation.

International conventions

The health facility should not allow distribution of free or low-cost suplies or products within the scope of the International Code of Marketing of Breast Milk Substitutes. It should also be tobacco free and support a tobacco-free environment.

Workplace and administrative procedures

A3

Standard precautions and cleanliness

A4

STANDARD PRECAUTIONS AND CLEANLINESS

Observe these precautions to protect the woman and her baby, and you as the health provider, from infections with bacteria and viruses, including HIV.

Wash hands

- Wash hands with soap and water:
  - Before and after caring for a woman or newborn, and before any treatment procedure.
  - Whenever the hands (or any other skin area) are contaminated with blood or other body fluids.
  - After removing the gloves, because they may have holes.
  - After changing soiled bedsheets or clothing.
- Keep nails short.

Wear gloves

- Wear sterile gloves when performing vaginal examination, delivery, cord cutting, repair of episiotomy or tear, blood drawing.
- Wear long sterile gloves for manual removal of placenta.
- Wear clean gloves when:
  - Handling and cleaning instruments
  - Handling contaminated waste
  - Cleaning blood and body fluid spills.
- Drawing blood.

Protect yourself from blood and other body fluids during deliveries

- Wear gloves; cover any cuts, abrasions or broken skin with a waterproof bandage; take care when handling any sharp instruments (use good light); and practice safe sharps disposal.
- Wear a long apron made from plastic or other fluid resistant material, and shoes.
- Protect your eyes and mouth from splashes of blood.

Practice safe sharps disposal

- Keep a puncture resistant container nearby.
- Use each needle and syringe only once.
- Do not recap, bend or break needles after giving an injection.
- Drop all used (disposable) needles, plastic syringes and blades directly into this container, without recapping, and without passing to another person.
- Empty or send for incineration when the container is three-quarters full.

Practice safe waste disposal

- Dispose of placenta or blood, or body fluid contaminated items, in leak-proof containers.
- Burn or bury contaminated solid waste.
- Wash hands, gloves and containers after disposal of infectious waste.
- Pour liquid waste down a drain or flushable toilet.

Deal with contaminated laundry

- Collect clothing or sheets stained with blood or body fluids and keep them separately from other laundry, wearing gloves or use a plastic bag. **DO NOT** touch them directly.
- Rinse off blood or other body fluids before washing with soap.

Sterilize and clean contaminated equipment

- Make sure that instruments which penetrate the skin (such as needles) are adequately sterilized, or that single-use instruments are disposed of after one use.
- Thoroughly clean or disinfect any equipment which comes into contact with intact skin (according to instructions).
- Use bleach for cleaning bowls and buckets, and for blood or body fluid spills.

Clean and disinfect gloves

- Reusing gloves is NOT recommended. If it is necessary to reuse gloves because the supply in the health facility is limited, clean and disinfect them.
- Wash the gloves in soap and water.
- Check for damage: Blow gloves full of air, twist the cuff closed, then hold under clean water and look for air leaks. Discard if damaged.
- Soak overnight in bleach solution with 0.5% available chlorine (made by adding 90 ml water to 10 ml bleach containing 5% available chlorine).
- Dry away from direct sunlight.
- Dust inside with talcum powder or starch.

This produces **disinfected** gloves. They are not sterile.

Sterilize gloves

- Sterilize by autoclaving.

PRINCIPLES OF GOOD CARE

ORGANIZING A VISIT

Receive and respond immediately

Receive every woman and newborn baby seeking care immediately after arrival (or organize reception by another provider).

- Perform Quick Check on all new incoming women and babies and those in the waiting room, especially if no-one is receiving them `B2`.
- At the first emergency sign on Quick Check, begin emergency assessment and management (RAM) `B1-B7` for the woman, or examine the newborn `J1-J11`.
- If she is in labour, accompany her to an appropriate place and follow the steps as in *Childbirth: labour, delivery and immediate postpartum care* `D1-D29`.
- If she has priority signs, examine her immediately using *Antenatal care*, *Postpartum* or *Post-abortion* care charts `C1-C19`, `E1-E10`, `B18-B22`.
- If no emergency or priority sign on RAM or not in labour, invite her to wait in the waiting room.
- If baby is newly born, looks small, examine immediately. Do not let the mother wait in the queue.

Begin each emergency care visit

- Introduce yourself.
- Ask the name of the woman.
- Encourage the companion to stay with the woman.
- Explain all procedures, ask permission, and keep the woman informed as much as you can about what you are doing. If she is unconscious, talk to the companion.
- Ensure and respect privacy during examination and discussion.
- If she came with a baby and the baby is well, ask the companion to take care of the baby during the maternal examination and treatment.

Care of woman or baby referred for special care to secondary level facility

- When a woman or baby is referred to a secondary level care facility because of a specific problem or complications, the underlying assumption of the Guide is that, at referral level, the woman/baby will be assessed, treated, counselled and advised on follow-up for that particular condition/ complication.
- Follow-up for that specific condition will be either:
  → organized by the referral facility or
  → written instructions will be given to the woman/baby for the skilled attendant at the primary level who referred the woman/baby
  → the woman/baby will be advised to go for a follow-up visit within 2 weeks according to severity of the condition.
- Routine care continues at the primary care level where it was initiated.

Begin each routine visit (for the woman and/or the baby)

- Greet the woman and offer her a seat.
- Introduce yourself.
- Ask her name (and the name of the baby).
- Ask her:
  → Why did you come? For yourself or for your baby?
  → For a scheduled (routine) visit?
  → For specific complaints about you or your baby?
  → First or follow-up visit?
  → Do you want to include your companion or other family member (parent if adolescent) in the examination and discussion?
- If the woman is recently delivered, assess the baby or ask to see the baby if not with the mother.
- If antenatal care, always revise the birth plan at the end of the visit after completing the chart.
- For a postpartum visit, if she came with the baby, also examine the baby:
  → Follow the appropriate charts according to pregnancy status/age of the baby and purpose of visit
  → Follow all steps on the chart and in relevant boxes.
- Unless the condition of the woman or the baby requires urgent referral to hospital, give preventive measures if due even if the woman has a condition "in yellow" that requires special treatment.

- If follow-up visit is within a week, and if no other complaints:
  → Assess the woman for the specific condition requiring follow-up only
  → Compare with earlier assessment and re-classify.
- If a follow-up visit is more than a week after the initial examination (but not the next scheduled visit):
  → Repeat the whole assessment as required for an antenatal, post-abortion, postpartum or newborn visit according to the schedule
  → If antenatal visit, revise the birth plan.

During the visit

- Explain all procedures.
- Ask permission before undertaking an examination or test.
- Keep the woman informed throughout. Discuss findings with her (and her partner).
- Ensure privacy during the examination and discussion.

At the end of the visit

- Ask the woman if she has any questions.
- Summarize the most important messages with her.
- Encourage her to return for a routine visit (tell her when) and if she has any concerns.
- Fill the Home-Based Maternal Record (HBMR) and give her the appropriate information sheet.
- Ask her if there are any points which need to be discussed and would she like support for this.

PRINCIPLES OF GOOD CARE

Organizing a visit

A5

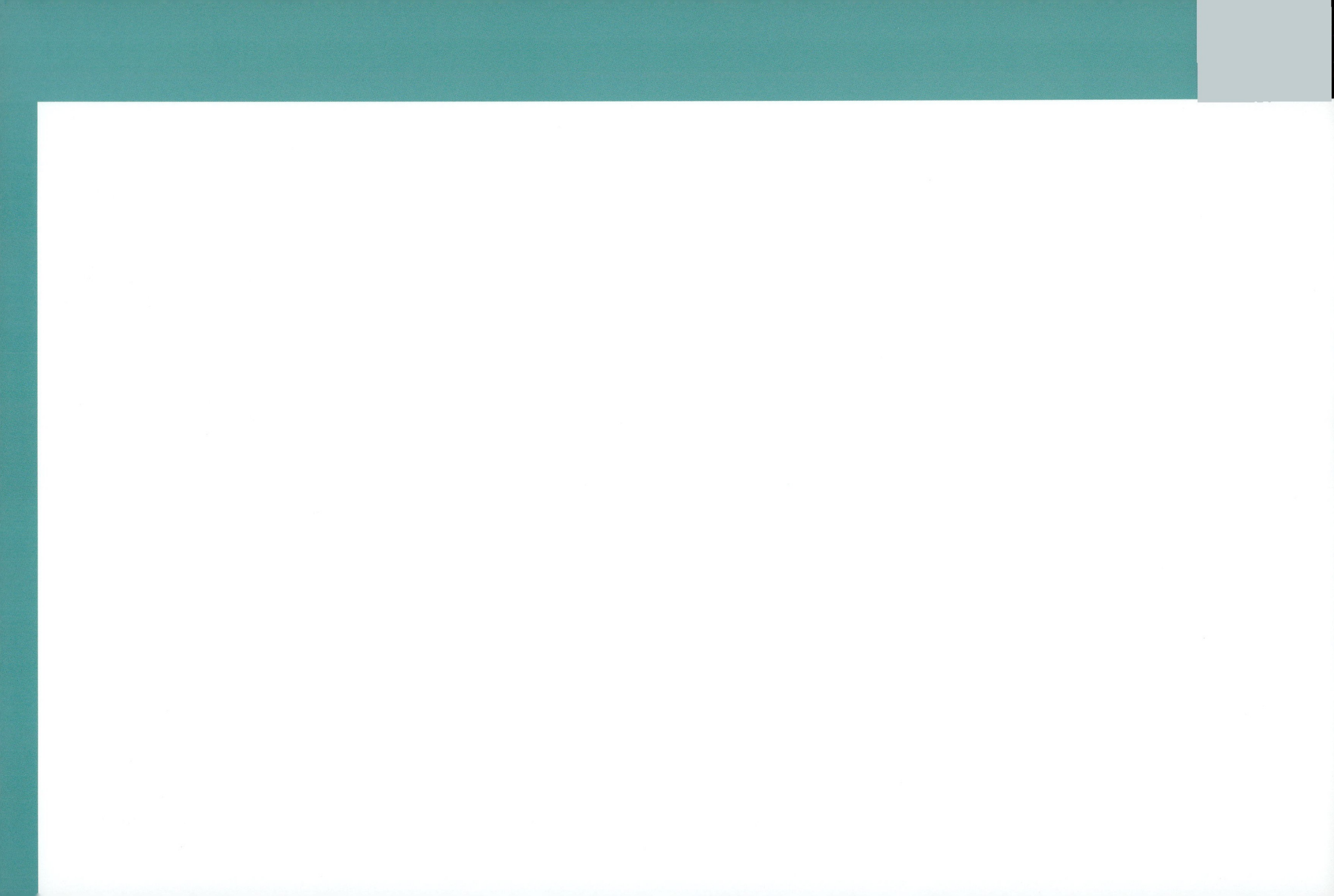

QUICK CHECK, RAPID ASSESSMENT AND MANAGEMENT OF WOMEN OF CHILDBEARING AGE

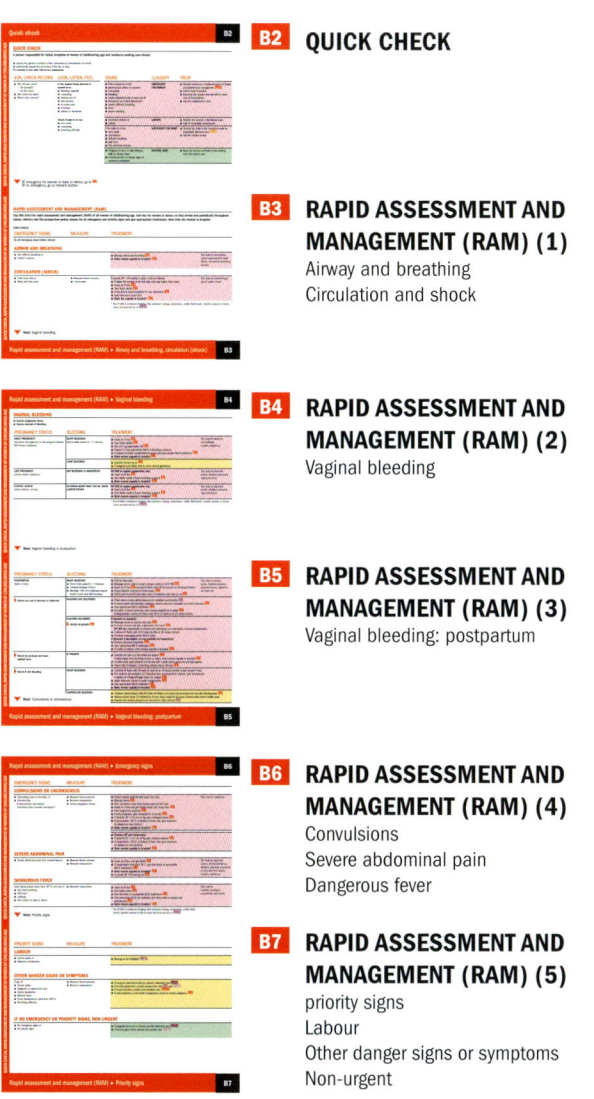

B2 QUICK CHECK

B3 RAPID ASSESSMENT AND MANAGEMENT (RAM) (1)
Airway and breathing
Circulation and shock

B4 RAPID ASSESSMENT AND MANAGEMENT (RAM) (2)
Vaginal bleeding

B5 RAPID ASSESSMENT AND MANAGEMENT (RAM) (3)
Vaginal bleeding: postpartum

B6 RAPID ASSESSMENT AND MANAGEMENT (RAM) (4)
Convulsions
Severe abdominal pain
Dangerous fever

B7 RAPID ASSESSMENT AND MANAGEMENT (RAM) (5)
priority signs
Labour
Other danger signs or symptoms
Non-urgent

- Perform Quick check immediately after the woman arrives **B2**.
  If any danger sign is seen, help the woman and send her quickly to the emergency room.

- Always begin a clinical visit with Rapid assessment and management (RAM) **B3-B7**:
  → Check for emergency signs first **B3-B6**.
    If present, provide emergency treatment and refer the woman urgently to hospital.
    Complete the referral form **N2**.
  → Check for priority signs. If present, manage according to charts **B7**.
  → If no emergency or priority signs, allow the woman to wait in line for routine care, according to pregnancy status.

Quick check, rapid assessment and management of women of childbearing age   **B1**

Quick check

B2

QUICK CHECK

A person responsible for initial reception of women of childbearing age and newborns seeking care should:

- assess the general condition of the careseeker(s) immediately on arrival
- periodically repeat this procedure if the line is long.

If a woman is very sick, talk to her companion.

ASK, CHECK RECORD	LOOK, LISTEN, FEEL	SIGNS	CLASSIFY	TREAT

■ Why did you come?
  → for yourself?
  → for the baby?
■ How old is the baby?
■ What is the concern?
	Is the woman being wheeled or carried in or:
	■ bleeding vaginally
	■ convulsing
	■ looking very ill
	■ unconscious
	■ in severe pain
	■ in labour
	■ delivery is imminent
	
	Check if baby is or has:
	■ very small
	■ convulsing
	■ breathing difficulty
		If the woman is or has:
		■ unconscious (does not answer)
		■ convulsing
		■ bleeding
		■ severe abdominal pain or looks very ill
		■ headache and visual disturbance
		■ severe difficulty breathing
		■ fever
		■ severe vomiting.
			EMERGENCY FOR WOMAN	■ Transfer woman to a treatment room for Rapid assessment and management B3-B7.
				■ Call for help if needed.
				■ Reassure the woman that she will be taken care of immediately.
				■ Ask her companion to stay.

		■ Imminent delivery or ■ Labour	**LABOUR**	■ Transfer the woman to the labour ward. ■ Call for immediate assessment.
		If the baby is or has: ■ very small ■ convulsions ■ difficult breathing ■ Heavy hypotonia ■ Hypothermia (moderate <36°C; severe <32°C). ■ just born ■ any maternal concern.	**EMERGENCY FOR BABY**	■ Transfer the baby to the treatment room for immediate Newborn care J1-J11. ■ Ask the mother to stay.
		■ Pregnant woman, or after delivery, with no danger signs ■ A newborn with no danger signs or maternal complaints.	**ROUTINE CARE**	■ Keep the woman and baby in the waiting room for routine care.

IF emergency for woman or baby or labour, go to B3.
IF no emergency, go to relevant section

RAPID ASSESSMENT AND MANAGEMENT (RAM)

Use this chart for rapid assessment and management (RAM) of all women of childbearing age, and also for women in labour, on first arrival and periodically throughout labour, delivery and the postpartum period. Assess for all emergency and priority signs and give appropriate treatments, then refer the woman to hospital.

FIRST ASSESS

EMERGENCY SIGNS	MEASURE	TREATMENT	
Do all emergency steps before referral			
AIRWAY AND BREATHING			
■ Very difficult breathing or ■ Central cyanosis		■ Manage airway and breathing `B9`. ■ **Refer woman urgently to hospital*** `B17`.	*This may be pneumonia, severe anaemia with heart failure, obstructed breathing, asthma.*
CIRCULATION (SHOCK)			
■ Cold moist skin or ■ Weak and fast pulse	■ Measure blood pressure ■ Count pulse	If systolic BP < 90 mmHg or pulse >110 per minute: ■ Position the woman on her left side with legs higher than chest. ■ Insert an IV line `B9`. ■ Give fluids rapidly `B9`. ■ If not able to insert peripheral IV, use alternative `B9`. ■ Keep her warm (cover her). ■ **Refer her urgently to hospital*** `B17`.	*This may be haemorrhagic shock, septic shock.*

* But if birth is imminent (bulging, thin perineum during contractions, visible fetal head), transfer woman to labour room and proceed as on `D1-D28`.

 Next: Vaginal bleeding

Rapid assessment and management (RAM) ▶ Airway and breathing, circulation (shock)   **B3**

Rapid assessment and management (RAM) ▶ Vaginal bleeding

B4

VAGINAL BLEEDING

- Assess pregnancy status
- Assess amount of bleeding

PREGNANCY STATUS	BLEEDING	TREATMENT	
EARLY PREGNANCY not aware of pregnancy, or not pregnant (uterus NOT above umbilicus)	**HEAVY BLEEDING** Pad or cloth soaked in < 5 minutes.	■ Insert an IV line **B9**. ■ Give fluids rapidly **B9**. ■ Give 0.2 mg ergometrine IM **B10**. ■ Repeat 0.2 mg ergometrine IM/IV if bleeding continues. ■ If suspect possible complicated abortion, give appropriate IM/IV antibiotics **B15**. ■ **Refer woman urgently to hospital B17**.	This may be abortion, menorrhagia, ectopic pregnancy.
	LIGHT BLEEDING	■ Examine woman as on **B19**. ■ If pregnancy not likely, refer to other clinical guidelines.	
LATE PREGNANCY (uterus above umbilicus)	**ANY BLEEDING IS DANGEROUS**	**DO NOT do vaginal examination, but:** ■ Insert an IV line **B9**. ■ Give fluids rapidly if heavy bleeding or shock **B3**. ■ **Refer woman urgently to hospital* B17**.	This may be placenta previa, abruptio placentae, ruptured uterus.
DURING LABOUR before delivery of baby	**BLEEDING MORE THAN 100 ML SINCE LABOUR BEGAN**	**DO NOT do vaginal examination, but:** ■ Insert an IV line **B9**. ■ Give fluids rapidly if heavy bleeding or shock **B3**. ■ **Refer woman urgently to hospital* B17**.	This may be placenta previa, abruptio placenta, ruptured uterus.

* But if birth is imminent (bulging, thin perineum during contractions, visible fetal head), transfer woman to labour room and proceed as on **D1-D28**.

▼ **Next:** Vaginal bleeding in postpartum

PREGNANCY STATUS	BLEEDING	TREATMENT	
POSTPARTUM (baby is born)	**HEAVY BLEEDING** ■ Pad or cloth soaked in < 5 minutes ■ Constant trickling of blood ■ Bleeding >250 ml or delivered outside health centre and still bleeding	■ Call for extra help. ■ Massage uterus until it is hard and give oxytocin 10 IU IM `B10`. ■ Insert an IV line `B9` and give IV fluids with 20 IU oxytocin at 60 drops/minute. ■ Empty bladder. Catheterize if necessary `B12`. ■ Check and record BP and pulse every 15 minutes and treat as on `B3`.	*This may be uterine atony, retained placenta, ruptured uterus, vaginal or cervical tear.*
▶ Check and ask if placenta is delivered	**PLACENTA NOT DELIVERED**	■ When uterus is hard, deliver placenta by controlled cord traction `D12`. ■ If unsuccessful and bleeding continues, remove placenta manually and check placenta `B11`. ■ Give appropriate IM/IV antibiotics `B15`. ■ If unable to remove placenta, refer woman urgently to hospital `B17`. During transfer, continue IV fluids with 20 IU of oxytocin at 30 drops/minute.	
	PLACENTA DELIVERED ▶ CHECK PLACENTA `B11`	**If placenta is complete:** ■ Massage uterus to express any clots `B10`. ■ If uterus remains soft, give ergometrine 0.2 mg IV `B10`. **DO NOT** give ergometrine to women with eclampsia, pre-eclampsia or known hypertension. ■ Continue IV fluids with 20 IU oxytocin/litre at 30 drops/minute. ■ Continue massaging uterus till it is hard. **If placenta is incomplete (or not available for inspection):** ■ Remove placental fragments `B11`. ■ Give appropriate IM/IV antibiotics `B15`. ■ If unable to remove, refer woman urgently to hospital `B17`.	
▶ Check for perineal and lower vaginal tears	**IF PRESENT**	■ Examine the tear and determine the degree `B12`. If third degree tear (involving rectum or anus), refer woman urgently to hospital `B17`. ■ For other tears: apply pressure over the tear with a sterile pad or gauze and put legs together. ■ Check after 5 minutes, if bleeding persists repair the tear `B12`.	
▶ Check if still bleeding	**HEAVY BLEEDING**	■ Continue IV fluids with 20 units of oxytocin at 30 drops/minute. Insert second IV line. ■ If IV oxytocin not available or if bleeding does not respond to oxytocin, give misoprostol, 4 tablets of 200µg (800µg) under the tongue `B10`. ■ Apply bimanual uterine or aortic compression `B10`. ■ Give appropriate IM/IV antibiotics `B15`. ■ **Refer woman urgently to hospital** `B17`.	
	CONTROLLED BLEEDING	■ Continue oxytocin infusion with 20 IU/litre of IV fluids at 20 drops/min for at least one hour after bleeding stops `B10`. ■ Observe closely (every 30 minutes) for 4 hours. Keep nearby for 24 hours. If severe pallor, refer to health centre. ■ Examine the woman using *Assess the mother after delivery* `D12`.	

▼ **Next:** Convulsions or unconscious

Rapid assessment and management (RAM) ▶ Emergency signs

B6

EMERGENCY SIGNS	MEASURE	TREATMENT	
CONVULSIONS OR UNCONSCIOUS			
■ Convulsing (now or recently), or ■ Unconscious If unconscious, ask relative "has there been a recent convulsion?"	■ Measure blood pressure ■ Measure temperature ■ Assess pregnancy status	■ Protect woman from fall and injury. Get help. ■ Manage airway **B9**. ■ After convulsion ends, help woman onto her left side. ■ Insert an IV line and give fluids slowly (30 drops/min) **B9**. ■ Give magnesium sulphate **B13**. ■ If early pregnancy, give diazepam IV or rectally **B14**. ■ If diastolic BP >110 mm of Hg, give antihypertensive **B14**. ■ If temperature >38°C, or history of fever, also give treatment for dangerous fever (below). ■ **Refer woman urgently to hospital* B17**.	*This may be eclampsia.*
		■ **Measure BP and temperature** ■ If diastolic BP >110 mm of Hg, give antihypertensive **B14**. ■ If temperature >38°C, or history of fever, also give treatment for dangerous fever (below). ■ **Refer woman urgently to hospital* B17**.	
SEVERE ABDOMINAL PAIN			
■ Severe abdominal pain (not normal labour)	■ Measure blood pressure ■ Measure temperature	■ Insert an IV line and give fluids **B9**. ■ If temperature more than 38°C, give first dose of appropriate IM/IV antiobiotics **B15**. ■ **Refer woman urgently to hospital* B17**. ■ If systolic BP <90 mm Hg see **B3**.	*This may be ruptured uterus, obstructed labour, abruptio placenta, puerperal or post-abortion sepsis, ectopic pregnancy.*
DANGEROUS FEVER			
Fever (temperature more than 38°C) and any of: ■ Very fast breathing ■ Stiff neck ■ Lethargy ■ Very weak/not able to stand	■ Measure temperature	■ Insert an IV line **B9**. ■ Give fluids slowly **B9**. ■ Give first dose of appropriate IM/IV antibiotics **B15**. ■ Give artesunate IM (if not available, give artemether or quinine IM) and glucose **B16**. ■ **Refer woman urgently to hospital* B17**.	*This may be malaria, meningitis, pneumonia, septicemia.*

▼ **Next:** Priority signs

* But if birth is imminent (bulging, thin perineum during contractions, visible fetal head), transfer woman to labour room and proceed as on **D1-D28**.

PRIORITY SIGNS	MEASURE	TREATMENT

LABOUR

- Labour pains or
- Ruptured membranes

- Manage as for Childbirth `D1-D28`.

OTHER DANGER SIGNS OR SYMPTOMS

If any of:
- Severe pallor
- Epigastric or abdominal pain
- Severe headache
- Blurred vision
- Fever (temperature more than 38°C)
- Breathing difficulty

- Measure blood pressure
- Measure temperature

- If pregnant (and not in labour), provide antenatal care `C1-C19`.
- If recently given birth, provide postpartum care `D21`. and `E1-E10`.
- If recent abortion, provide post-abortion care `B20-B21`.
- If early pregnancy, or not aware of pregnancy, check for ectopic pregnancy `B19`.

IF NO EMERGENCY OR PRIORITY SIGNS, NON URGENT

- No emergency signs or
- No priority signs

- If pregnant (and not in labour), provide antenatal care `C1-C19`.
- If recently given birth, provide postpartum care `E1-E10`.

Rapid assessment and management (RAM) ▶ Priority signs

Emergency treatments for the woman

EMERGENCY TREATMENTS FOR THE WOMAN

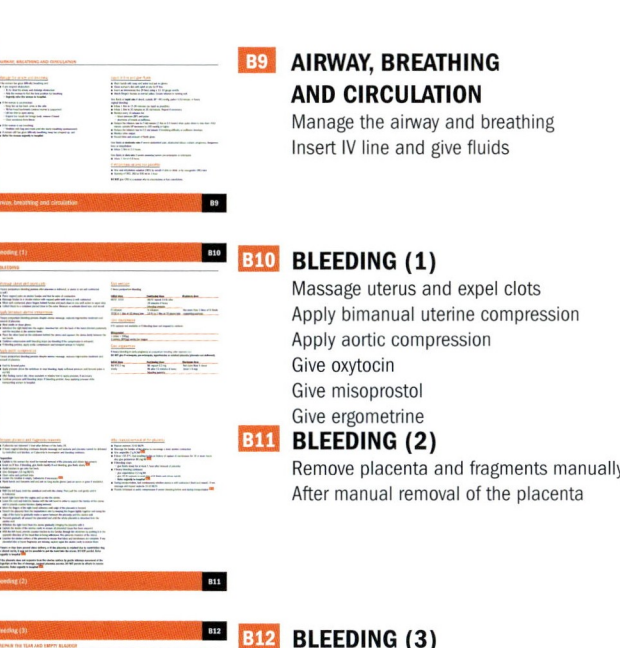

B9 AIRWAY, BREATHING AND CIRCULATION
Manage the airway and breathing
Insert IV line and give fluids

B10 BLEEDING (1)
Massage uterus and expel clots
Apply bimanual uterine compression
Apply aortic compression
Give oxytocin
Give misoprostol
Give ergometrine

B11 BLEEDING (2)
Remove placenta and fragments manually
After manual removal of the placenta

B12 BLEEDING (3)
Repair the tear
Empty bladder

B13 ECLAMPSIA AND PRE-ECLAMPSIA (1)
Important considerations in caring for a woman with eclampsia and pre-eclampsia
Give magnesium sulphate

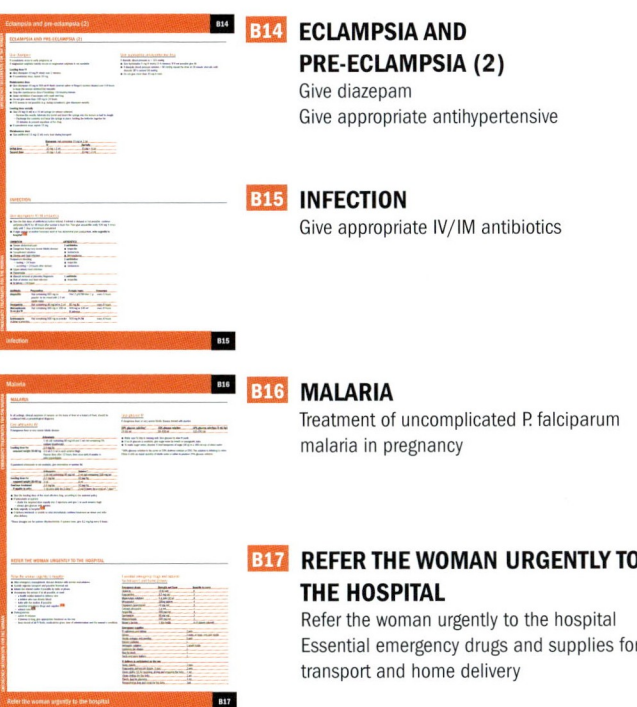

B14 ECLAMPSIA AND PRE-ECLAMPSIA (2)
Give diazepam
Give appropriate antihypertensive

B15 INFECTION
Give appropriate IV/IM antibiotics

B16 MALARIA
Treatment of uncomplicated P. falciparum malaria in pregnancy

B17 REFER THE WOMAN URGENTLY TO THE HOSPITAL
Refer the woman urgently to the hospital
Essential emergency drugs and supplies for transport and home delivery

- This section has details on emergency treatments identified during Rapid assessment and management (RAM) **B3-B6** to be given before referral.
- Give the treatment and refer the woman urgently to hospital **B17**.
- If drug treatment, give the first dose of the drugs before referral. Do not delay referral by giving non-urgent treatments.

AIRWAY, BREATHING AND CIRCULATION

Manage the airway and breathing

If the woman has great difficulty breathing and:
- If you suspect obstruction:
  → Try to clear the airway and dislodge obstruction
  → Help the woman to find the best position for breathing
  → **Urgently refer the woman to hospital.**

- If the woman is unconscious:
  → Keep her on her back, arms at the side
  → Tilt her head backwards (unless trauma is suspected)
  → Lift her chin to open airway
  → Inspect her mouth for foreign body; remove if found
  → Clear secretions from throat.

- If the woman is not breathing:
  → Ventilate with bag and mask until she starts breathing spontaneously
- If woman still has great difficulty breathing, keep her propped up, and
- **Refer the woman urgently to hospital.**

Insert IV line and give fluids

- Wash hands with soap and water and put on gloves.
- Clean woman's skin with spirit at site for IV line.
- Insert an intravenous line (IV line) using a 16-18 gauge needle.
- Attach Ringer's lactate or normal saline. Ensure infusion is running well.

Give fluids at **rapid rate** if shock, systolic BP <90 mmHg, pulse>110/minute, or heavy vaginal bleeding:
- Infuse 1 litre in 15-20 minutes (as rapid as possible).
- Infuse 1 litre in 30 minutes at 30 ml/minute. Repeat if necessary.
- Monitor every 15 minutes for:
  → blood pressure (BP) and pulse
  → shortness of breath or puffiness.
- Reduce the infusion rate to 3 ml/minute (1 litre in 6-8 hours) when pulse slows to less than 100/minute, systolic BP increases to 100 mmHg or higher.
- Reduce the infusion rate to 0.5 ml/minute if breathing difficulty or puffiness develops.
- Monitor urine output.
- Record time and amount of fluids given.

Give fluids at **moderate rate** if severe abdominal pain, obstructed labour, ectopic pregnancy, dangerous fever or dehydration:
- Infuse 1 litre in 2-3 hours.

Give fluids at **slow rate** if severe anaemia/severe pre-eclampsia or eclampsia:
- Infuse 1 litre in 6-8 hours.

If intravenous access not possible

- Give oral rehydration solution (ORS) by mouth if able to drink, or by nasogastric (NG) tube.
- Quantity of ORS: 300 to 500 ml in 1 hour.

DO NOT give ORS to a woman who is unconscious or has convulsions.

Bleeding (1)　　　　　　　　　　　　　　　　　　　　　　　　　　　B10

EMERGENCY TREATMENTS FOR THE WOMAN

BLEEDING

Massage uterus and expel clots

If heavy postpartum bleeding persists after placenta is delivered, or uterus is not well contracted (is soft):
- Place cupped palm on uterine fundus and feel for state of contraction.
- Massage fundus in a circular motion with cupped palm until uterus is well contracted.
- When well contracted, place fingers behind fundus and push down in one swift action to expel clots.
- Collect blood in a container placed close to the vulva. Measure or estimate blood loss, and record.

Apply bimanual uterine compression

If heavy postpartum bleeding persists despite uterine massage, oxytocin/ergometrine treatment and removal of placenta:
- Wear sterile gloves.
- Introduce the right hand into the vagina, clenched fist, with the back of the hand directed posteriorly and the knuckles in the anterior fornix.
- Place the other hand on the abdomen behind the uterus and squeeze the uterus firmly between the two hands.
- Continue compression until bleeding stops (no bleeding if the compression is released).
- If bleeding persists, apply aortic compression and transport woman to hospital.

Apply aortic compression

If heavy postpartum bleeding persists despite uterine massage, oxytocin/ergometrine treatment and removal of placenta:
- Feel for femoral pulse.
- Apply pressure above the umbilicus to stop bleeding. Apply sufficient pressure until femoral pulse is not felt.
- After finding correct site, show assistant or relative how to apply pressure, if necessary.
- Continue pressure until bleeding stops. If bleeding persists, keep applying pressure while transporting woman to hospital.

Give oxytocin

If heavy postpartum bleeding

Initial dose	Continuing dose	Maximum dose
IM/IV: 10 IU	IM/IV: repeat 10 IU after 20 minutes if heavy bleeding persists	
IV infusion: 20 IU in 1 litre at 60 drops/min	IV infusion: 10 IU in 1 litre at 30 drops/min	Not more than 3 litres of IV fluids containing oxytocin

Give misoprostol

If IV oxytocin not available or if bleeding does not respond to oxytocin.

Misoprostol
1 tablet = 200µg
4 tablets (800µg) under the tongue

Give ergometrine

If heavy bleeding in early pregnancy or postpartum bleeding (after oxytocin) but
DO NOT give if eclampsia, pre-eclampsia, hypertension or retained placenta (placenta not delivered).

Initial dose	Continuing dose	Maximum dose
IM/IV: 0.2 mg slowly	IM: repeat 0.2 mg IM after 15 minutes if heavy bleeding persists	Not more than 5 doses (total 1.0 mg)

Remove placenta and fragments manually

- If placenta not delivered 1 hour after delivery of the baby, OR.
- If heavy vaginal bleeding continues despite massage and oxytocin and placenta cannot be delivered by controlled cord traction, or if placenta is incomplete and bleeding continues.

Preparation
- Explain to the woman the need for manual removal of the placenta and obtain her consent.
- Insert an IV line. If bleeding, give fluids rapidly. If not bleeding, give fluids slowly B9.
- Assist woman to get onto her back.
- Give diazepam (10 mg IM/IV).
- Clean vulva and perineal area.
- Ensure the bladder is empty. Catheterize if necessary B12.
- Wash hands and forearms well and put on long sterile gloves (and an apron or gown if available).

Technique
- With the left hand, hold the umbilical cord with the clamp. Then pull the cord gently until it is horizontal.
- Insert right hand into the vagina and up into the uterus.
- Leave the cord and hold the fundus with the left hand in order to support the fundus of the uterus and to provide counter-traction during removal.
- Move the fingers of the right hand sideways until edge of the placenta is located.
- Detach the placenta from the implantation site by keeping the fingers tightly together and using the edge of the hand to gradually make a space between the placenta and the uterine wall.
- Proceed gradually all around the placental bed until the whole placenta is detached from the uterine wall.
- Withdraw the right hand from the uterus gradually, bringing the placenta with it.
- Explore the inside of the uterine cavity to ensure all placental tissue has been removed.
- With the left hand, provide counter-traction to the fundus through the abdomen by pushing it in the opposite direction of the hand that is being withdrawn. This prevents inversion of the uterus.
- Examine the uterine surface of the placenta to ensure that lobes and membranes are complete. If any placental lobe or tissue fragments are missing, explore again the uterine cavity to remove them.

If hours or days have passed since delivery, or if the placenta is retained due to constriction ring or closed cervix, it may not be possible to put the hand into the uterus. DO NOT persist. Refer urgently to hospital B17.

If the placenta does not separate from the uterine surface by gentle sideways movement of the fingertips at the line of cleavage, suspect placenta accreta. DO NOT persist in efforts to remove placenta. Refer urgently to hospital B17.

After manual removal of the placenta

- Repeat oxytocin 10-IU IM/IV.
- Massage the fundus of the uterus to encourage a tonic uterine contraction.
- Give antibiotic prophylaxis: a single dose of ampicillin 2 g IV/IM B15.
- If fever >38.5°C, foul-smelling lochia or history of rupture of membranes for 18 or more hours, give clindamycin 600 mg IV every six to eight hours, and gentamycin 1-1.5 mg/kg or 60-80 mg IV every eight hours (antibiotic should continue for at least 24-48 hours after complete resolution of clinical signs and symptoms). B15.
- If bleeding stops:
  → give fluids slowly for at least 1 hour after removal of placenta.
- If heavy bleeding continues:
  → give ergometrine 0.2 mg IM
  → give 20 IU oxytocin in each litre of IV fluids and infuse rapidly
  → **Refer urgently to hospital B17.**
- During transportation, feel continuously whether uterus is well contracted (hard and round). If not, massage and repeat oxytocin 10 IU IM/IV.
- Provide bimanual or aortic compression if severe bleeding before and during transportation B10.

Bleeding (2)

Bleeding (3) — B12

REPAIR THE TEAR AND EMPTY BLADDER

Repair the tear or episiotomy

- Examine the tear and determine the degree:
  → The tear is small and involved only vaginal mucosa and connective tissues and underlying muscles (first or second degree tear). If the tear is not bleeding, leave the wound open
  → The tear is long and deep through the perineum and involves the anal sphincter and rectal mucosa (third and fourth degree tear). Cover it with a clean pad and **refer the woman urgently to hospital** B17.
- If first or second degree tear and heavy bleeding persists after applying pressure over the wound:
  → Suture the tear or refer for suturing if no one is available with suturing skills
  → Suture the tear using universal precautions, aseptic technique and sterile equipment
  → Use local infiltration with lidocaine
  → Use a needle holder and a 21 gauge, 4 cm, curved needle
  → Use absorbable polyglycol suture material
  → Make sure that the apex of the tear is reached before you begin suturing
  → Ensure that edges of the tear match up well
  → Provide emotional support and encouragement
  → **DO NOT** suture if more than 12 hours since delivery. **Refer woman to hospital.**

Empty bladder

If bladder is distended and the woman is unable to pass urine:
- Encourage the woman to urinate.
- If she is unable to urinate, catheterize the bladder:
  → Wash hands
  → Put on clean gloves
  → Clean urethral area with antiseptic
  → Spread labia. Clean area again
  → Insert catheter up to 4 cm
  → Measure urine and record amount
  → Remove catheter.

ECLAMPSIA AND PRE-ECLAMPSIA (1)

Give magnesium sulphate

If severe pre-eclampsia and eclampsia

IV/IM combined dose (loading dose)
- Insert IV line and give fluids slowly (normal saline or Ringer's lactate) — 1 litre in 6-8 hours (3 ml/minute) `B9`.
- Give 4 g of magnesium sulphate (20 ml of 20% solution) IV slowly over 20 minutes (woman may feel warm during injection).

AND:
- Give 10 g of magnesium sulphate IM: give 5 g (10 ml of 50% solution) IM deep in upper outer quadrant of each buttock with 1 ml of 2% lignocaine in the same syringe.

If unable to give IV, give IM only (loading dose)
- Give 10 g of magnesium sulphate IM: give 5 g (10 ml of 50% solution) IM deep in upper outer quadrant of each buttock with 1 ml of 2% lignocaine in the same syringe.

If convulsions recur
- After 15 minutes, give an additional 2 g of magnesium sulphate (10 ml of 20% solution) IV over 20 minutes. If convulsions still continue, give diazepam `B14`.

If referral delayed for long, or the woman is in late labour, continue treatment:
- Give 5 g of 50% magnesium sulphate solution IM with 1 ml of 2% lignocaine every 4 hours in alternate buttocks until 24 hours after birth or after last convulsion (whichever is later).
- Monitor urine output: collect urine and measure the quantity.
- Before giving the next dose of magnesium sulphate, ensure:
  → knee jerk is present
  → urine output >100 ml/4 hrs
  → respiratory rate >16/min.
- **DO NOT** give the next dose if any of these signs:
  → knee jerk absent
  → urine output <100 ml/4 hrs
  → respiratory rate <16/min.
- Record findings and drugs given.

Important considerations in caring for a woman with eclampsia or pre-eclampsia

- Do not leave the woman on her own.
  → Help her into the left side position and protect her from fall and injury
  → Place padded tongue blades between her teeth to prevent a tongue bite, and secure it to prevent aspiration (**DO NOT** attempt this during a convulsion).
- Give IV 20% magnesium sulphate slowly over 20 minutes. Rapid injection can cause respiratory failure or death.
  → If respiratory depression (breathing less than 16/minute) occurs after magnesium sulphate, do not give any more magnesium sulphate. Give the antidote: calcium gluconate 1 g IV (10 ml of 10% solution) over 10 minutes.
- **DO NOT** give intravenous fluids rapidly.
- **DO NOT** give intravenously 50% magnesium sulphate without diluting it to 20%.
- **Refer urgently to hospital** unless in late labour.
  → If delivery imminent, manage as in Childbirth `D1-D29` and accompany the woman during transport
  → Keep her in the left side position
  → If a convulsion occurs during the journey, give magnesium sulphate and protect her from fall and injury.

Formulation of magnesium sulphate

		50% solution: vial containing 5 g in 10 ml (1 g/2 ml)	20% solution: to make 10 ml of 20% solution, add 4 ml of 50% solution to 6 ml sterile water
IM	5 g	10 ml and 1 ml 2% lignocaine	Not applicable
IV	4 g	8 ml	20 ml
	2 g	4 ml	10 ml

After receiving magnesium sulphate a woman feel flushing, thirst, headache, nausea or may vomit.

Eclampsia and pre-eclampsia (2)

B14

EMERGENCY TREATMENTS FOR THE WOMAN

ECLAMPSIA AND PRE-ECLAMPSIA (2)

Give diazepam

If convulsions occur in early pregnancy or
If magnesium sulphate toxicity occurs or magnesium sulphate is not available.

Loading dose IV
- Give diazepam 10 mg IV slowly over 2 minutes.
- If convulsions recur, repeat 10 mg.

Maintenance dose
- Give diazepam 40 mg in 500 ml IV fluids (normal saline or Ringer's lactate) titrated over 6-8 hours to keep the woman sedated but rousable.
- Stop the maintenance dose if breathing <16 breaths/minute.
- Assist ventilation if necessary with mask and bag.
- Do not give more than 100 mg in 24 hours.
- If IV access is not possible (e.g. during convulsion), give diazepam rectally.

Loading dose rectally
- Give 20 mg (4 ml) in a 10 ml syringe (or urinary catheter):
  → Remove the needle, lubricate the barrel and insert the syringe into the rectum to half its length.
  → Discharge the contents and leave the syringe in place, holding the buttocks together for 10 minutes to prevent expulsion of the drug.
- If convulsions recur, repeat 10 mg.

Maintenance dose
- Give additional 10 mg (2 ml) every hour during transport.

Diazepam: vial containing 10 mg in 2 ml

	IV	Rectally
Initial dose	10 mg = 2 ml	20 mg = 4 ml
Second dose	10 mg = 2 ml	10 mg = 2 ml

Give appropriate antihypertensive drug

If diastolic blood pressure is > 110 mmHg:
- Give hydralazine 5 mg IV slowly (3-4 minutes). If IV not possible give IM.
- If diastolic blood pressure remains > 90 mmHg, repeat the dose at 30 minute intervals until diastolic BP is around 90 mmHg.
- Do not give more than 20 mg in total.

INFECTION

Give appropriate IV/IM antibiotics

- Give the first dose of antibiotic(s) before referral. If referral is delayed or not possible, continue antibiotics IM/IV for 48 hours after woman is fever free.
- If signs persist or mother becomes weak or has abdominal pain postpartum, **refer urgently to hospital** B17.

CONDITION	ANTIBIOTICS
■ Complicated abortion	**2 antibiotics** ■ Ampicillin ■ Gentamicin
■ Dangerous maternal fever/very severe febrile disease (e.g. postpartum endometritis)	**2 antibiotics**: ■ Clindamycin ■ Gentamicin
■ Manual removal of placenta/fragments ■ Risk of uterine and fetal infection	**1 antibiotic**: ■ Ampicillin or First-generation cephalosporin

Antibiotic	Preparation	Dosage/route	Frequency
Ampicillin	Vial containing 500 mg as powder: to be mixed with 2.5 ml sterile water	First 2 g IV/IM then 1 g	every 6 hours
Gentamicin	Vial containing 40 mg/ml in 2 ml	80 mg IM	every 8 hours
Cefazolin	Vial containing 1g (powder for injection / as sodium salt).	First: 1 g IV/IM	every 6 hours
Clindamycin	Vial containing 150 mg for injection (as phosphate)/ml Capsule: 150 mg (as hydrochloride).	150 mg IV/IM/PO.	every 6 – 8 hours

Infection

Malaria B16

MALARIA

Treatment of uncomplicated P. falciparum malaria in pregnancy

In all settings, clinical suspicion of malaria, on the basis of fever or a history of fever, should be confirmed with a parasitological diagnosis.

First trimester of pregnancy: Give Quinine + Clindamycin for 7 days.
- Quinine:
  - → Preparation: 2 ml vial containing 300 mg/ml.
  - → Loading dose (assumed weight 50-60 kg): 20 mg/kg.
  - → Continue treatment if unable to refer: 10 mg/kg (2 ml/8 hours).
  - → The required dosage is preferably diluted in a IV 5% glucose solution, to correct hypoglycaemia.

- Clindamycin B15.
- Administer oral quinine & clindamycin when the patient has recovered sufficiently to take tablets, to complete a total course of 7 days.

Second and third trimesters: Give Artesunate
- Preparation: 1 ml vial containing 60 mg/ml and 1 ml vial containing 5% bicarbonate solution.
- Dose: 2.4 mg/kg IM/IV at 0, 12 hours, 24 hours, THEN once daily, until oral artesunate 2 mg / kg / day can be taken, to complete a total course of 7 days.

Give the loading dose of the most effective drug.

Refer urgently to hospital B17.

If delivery imminent or unable to refer immediately, continue treatment as above and refer after delivery.

REFER THE WOMAN URGENTLY TO THE HOSPITAL

Refer the woman urgently to hospital

- After emergency management, discuss decision with woman and relatives.
- Quickly organize transport and possible financial aid.
- Inform the referral centre if possible by radio or phone.
- Accompany the woman if at all possible, or send:
  → a health worker trained in delivery care
  → a relative who can donate blood
  → baby with the mother, if possible
  → essential emergency drugs and supplies.
  → referral note N2.
- During journey:
  → watch IV infusion
  → if journey is long, give appropriate treatment on the way
  → keep record of all IV fluids, medications given, time of administration and the woman's condition.

Essential emergency drugs and supplies for transport and home delivery

Emergency drugs	Strength and Form	Quantity to carry
Oxytocin	10 IU vial	6
Ergometrine	0.2 mg vial	2
Magnesium sulphate	5 g vials (20 g)	4
Misoprostol	200µg tablets	4
Diazepam (parenteral)	10 mg vial	3
Calcium gluconate	1 g vial	1
Ampicillin	500 mg vial	4
Gentamicin	80 mg vial	3
Clindamycin	150 mg vial	3
Quinine	2 ml vial	3
Artesunate	60 mg vial	3
Ringer's lactate	1 litre bottle	4 (if distant referral)

Emergency supplies	
IV catheters and tubing	2 sets
Gloves	2 pairs, sterile
Sterile syringes and needles	5 sets
Urinary catheter	1
Antiseptic solution	1 small bottle
Container for sharps	1
Bag for trash	1
Torch and extra battery	1

If delivery is anticipated on the way	
Soap, towels	2 sets
Disposable delivery kit (blade, 3 ties)	2 sets
Clean cloths (3) for receiving, drying and wrapping the baby	1 set
Clean clothes for the baby	1 set
Plastic bag for placenta	1 set
Resuscitation bag and mask for the baby	1 set

Bleeding in early pregnancy and post-abortion care — B18

BLEEDING IN EARLY PREGNANCY AND POST-ABORTION CARE

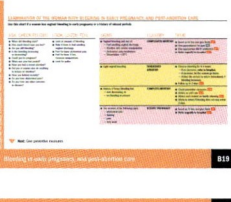

B19 EXAMINATION OF THE WOMAN WITH BLEEDING IN EARLY PREGNANCY AND POST-ABORTION CAR

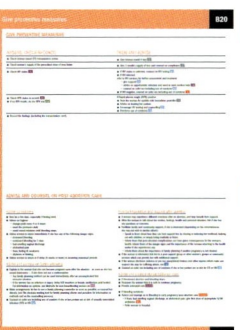

B20 GIVE PREVENTIVE MEASURES

B21 ADVISE AND COUNSEL ON POST-ABORTION CARE
Advise on self-care
Advise and counsel on family planning
Provide information and support after abortion
Advise and counsel during follow-up visits

- Always begin with Rapid assessment and management (RAM) B3-B7.
- Next use the Bleeding in early pregnancy/post abortion care B19 to assess the woman with light vaginal bleeding or a history of missed periods.
- Use chart on Preventive measures B20 to provide preventive measures due to all women.
- Use Advise and Counsel on post-abortion care B21 to advise on self care, danger signs, follow-up visit, family planning.
- Record all treatment given, positive findings, and the scheduled next visit in the home-based and clinic recording forms.
- If the woman is HIV positive, adolescent or has special needs, use G1-G11 H1-H4.

EXAMINATION OF THE WOMAN WITH BLEEDING IN EARLY PREGNANCY, AND POST-ABORTION CARE

Use this chart if a woman has vaginal bleeding in early pregnancy or a history of missed periods

ASK, CHECK RECORD
- When did bleeding start?
- How much blood have you lost?
- Are you still bleeding?
- Is the bleeding increasing or decreasing?
- Could you be pregnant?
- When was your last period?
- Have you had a recent abortion?
- Did you or anyone else do anything to induce an abortion?
- Have you fainted recently?
- Do you have abdominal pain?
- Do you have any other concerns to discuss?

LOOK, LISTEN, FEEL
- Look at amount of bleeding.
- Note if there is foul-smelling vaginal discharge.
- Feel for lower abdominal pain.
- Feel for fever. If hot, measure temperature.
- Look for pallor.
- Check pulse rate.
- Assess uterine size.

SIGNS	CLASSIFY	TREAT
■ Vaginal bleeding and any of: → Foul-smelling vaginal discharge → Abortion with uterine manipulation → Abdominal pain/tenderness → Temperature >38°C	COMPLICATED ABORTION	■ Insert an IV line and give fluids B9. ■ Give Ibuprofen for pain (tablets 400 mg – 600 mg). Dose: 600-1200 mg /day F4. ■ Give appropriate IM/IV antibiotics B15. ■ **Refer urgently to hospital** B17.
■ Light vaginal bleeding	THREATENED ABORTION	■ Observe bleeding for 4-6 hours: → - If no decrease or worsening in bleeding or vital signs, refer to hospital. **refer to hospital.** → If decrease, let the woman go home. → Advise the woman to return immediately if bleeding increases. ■ Follow up in 2 days B21.
■ History of heavy bleeding but: → now decreasing, or → no bleeding at present	COMPLETE ABORTION	■ Check preventive measures B20. ■ Advise on self-care B21. ■ Advise and counsel on family planning B21. ■ Advise to return if bleeding does not stop within 2 days.
■ Two or more of the following signs: → abdominal pain → fainting → pale → very weak	ECTOPIC PREGNANCY	■ Insert an IV line and give fluids B9. ■ **Refer urgently to hospital** B17.

 Next: Give preventive measures

Bleeding in early pregnancy, and post-abortion care

B19

Give preventive measures

B20

BLEEDING IN EARLY PREGNANCY AND POST-ABORTION CARE

GIVE PREVENTIVE MEASURES

ASSESS, CHECK RECORDS	TREAT AND ADVISE
■ Check tetanus toxoid (TT) immunization status.	■ Give tetanus toxoid if due **F2**.
■ Check woman's supply of the prescribed dose of iron/folate.	■ Give 3 month's supply of iron and counsel on compliance **F3**.
■ Check HIV status **C6**.	■ If HIV status is unknown, counsel on HIV testing **G3**. ■ If HIV-infected: refer to HIV services for further assessment and treatment → give support **G4** → advise on opportunistic infection and need to seek medical help **C10** → counsel on safer sex including use of condoms **G2**. ■ If HIV-negative, counsel on safer sex including use of condoms **G4**.
■ Check RPR status in records **C5**. ■ If no RPR results, do the RPR test **L5**.	If Rapid plasma reagin (RPR) positive: ■ Treat the woman for syphilis with benzathine penicillin **F6**. ■ Advise on treating her partner. ■ Encourage HIV testing and counselling **G3**. ■ Reinforce use of condoms **G2**.
■ Record the findings (including the immunization card).	

ADVISE AND COUNSEL ON POST-ABORTION CARE

Advise on self-care

- Rest for a few days, especially if feeling tired.
- Advise on hygiene
  - → change pads every 4 to 6 hours
  - → wash the perineum daily
  - → avoid sexual relations until bleeding stops.
- Advise woman to return immediately if she has any of the following danger signs:
  - → increased bleeding
  - → foul-smelling vaginal discharge
  - → abdominal pain
  - → fever, feeling ill, weakness
  - → dizziness or fainting.
- Advise woman to return in if delay (6 weeks or more) in resuming menstrual periods.

Advise and counsel on family planning

- Explain to the woman that she can become pregnant soon after the abortion - as soon as she has sexual intercourse — if she does not use a contraceptive:
  - → Any family planning method can be used immediately after an uncomplicated first trimester abortion.
  - → If the woman has an infection or injury: delay IUD insertion or female sterilization until healed. For information on options, see Methods for non-breastfeeding women on D27.
- Make arrangements for her to see a family planning counsellor as soon as possible, or counsel her directly. (see The decision-making tool for family planning clients and providers for information on methods and on the counselling process).
- Counsel on safer sex including use of condom if she or her partner are at risk of sexually transmitted infection (STI) or HIV G2.

Provide information and support after abortion

- A woman may experience different emotions after an abortion, and may benefit from support:
- Allow the woman to talk about her worries, feelings, health and personal situation. Ask if she has any questions or concerns.
- Facilitate family and community support, if she is interested (depending on the circumstances, she may not wish to involve others).
  - → Speak to them about how they can best support her, by sharing or reducing her workload, helping out with children, or simply being available to listen.
  - → Inform them that post-abortion complications can have grave consequences for the woman's health. Inform them of the danger signs and the importance of the woman returning to the health worker if she experiences any.
  - → Inform them about the importance of family planning if another pregnancy is not desired.
- If the woman is interested, link her to a peer support group or other women's groups or community services which can provide her with additional support.
- If the woman discloses violence or you see unexplained bruises and other injuries which make you suspect she may be suffering abuse, see H4.

Advise and counsel during follow-up visits

- If threatened abortion and bleeding stops:
  - → Reassure the woman that it is safe to continue pregnancy.
  - → Provide antenatal care C1-C18.

- If bleeding continues:
- Assess and manage as in Bleeding in early pregnancy/post-abortion care B18-B22.
  - → If fever, foul-smelling vaginal discharge, or abdominal pain, give first dose of appropriate IV/IM antibiotics B15.
- Refer woman to hospital.

Antenatal care

ANTENATAL CARE

- Always begin with **Rapid assessment and management (RAM)** `B3-B7`. If the woman has no emergency or priority signs and has come for antenatal care, use this section for further care.

- Next use the **Pregnancy status and birth plan chart** `C2` to ask the woman about her present pregnancy status, history of previous pregancies, and check her for general danger signs. Decide on an appropriate place of birth for the woman using this chart and prepare the birth and emergency plan. The birth plan should be reviewed during every follow-up visit.

- Check all women for pre-eclampsia, anaemia, syphilis and HIV status according to the charts `C3-C6`.

- In cases where an abnormal sign is identified (volunteered or observed), use the charts **Respond to observed signs or volunteered problems** `C7-C11` to classify the condition and identify appropriate treatment(s).

- Give **preventive measures** due `C12`.

- Develop a **birth and emergency plan** `C14-C15`.

- Advise and counsel on nutrition `C13`, family planning `C16`, labour signs, danger signs `C15`, routine and follow-up visits `C17` using **Information and Counselling sheets** `M1-M19`.

- Record all positive findings, birth plan, treatments given and the next scheduled visit in the home-based maternal card/clinic recording form.

- Offer ART to all HIV-infected women `G9`.

Antenatal care

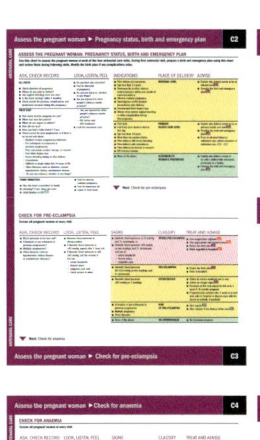

C2 ASSESS THE PREGNANT WOMAN: PREGNANCY STATUS, BIRTH AND EMERGENCY PLAN

C3 CHECK FOR PRE-ECLAMPSIA

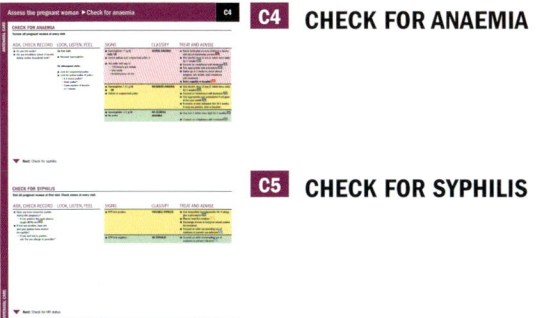

C4 CHECK FOR ANAEMIA

C5 CHECK FOR SYPHILIS

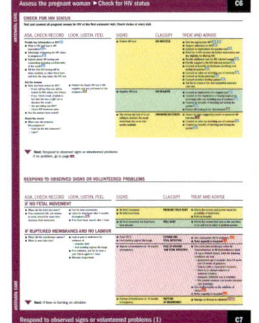

C6 CHECK FOR HIV STATUS

C7 RESPOND TO OBSERVED SIGNS OR VOLUNTEERED PROBLEMS (1)
If no fetal movement
If ruptured membrane and no labour

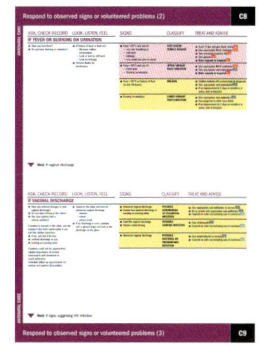

C8 RESPOND TO OBSERVED SIGNS OR VOLUNTEERED PROBLEMS (2)
If fever or burning on urination

C9 RESPOND TO OBSERVED SIGNS OR VOLUNTEERED PROBLEMS (3)
If vaginal discharge

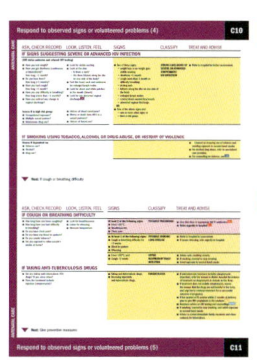

C10 RESPOND TO OBSERVED SIGNS OR VOLUNTEERED PROBLEMS (4)
If signs suggesting severe or advanced HIV infection
If smoking, alcohol or drug abuse, or history of violence

C11 RESPOND TO OBSERVED SIGNS OR VOLUNTEERED PROBLEMS (5)
If cough or breathing difficulty
If taking anti-tuberculosis drugs

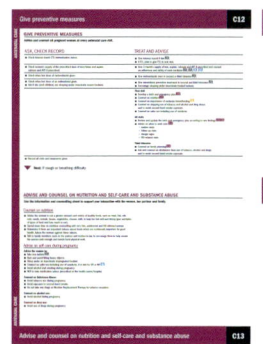

C12 GIVE PREVENTIVE MEASURES

C13 ADVISE AND COUNSEL ON NUTRITION AND SELF-CARE
Counsel on nutrition
Advise on self-care during pregnancy

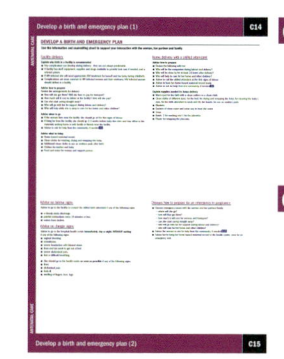

C14 DEVELOP A BIRTH AND EMERGENCY PLAN
Facility delivery
Home delivery with a skilled attendant

C15 Advise on labour signs
Advise on danger signs
Discuss how to prepare for an emergency in pregnancy

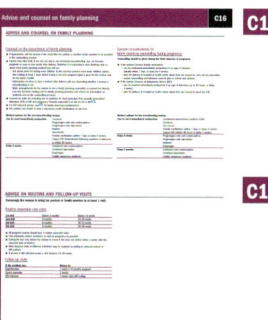

C16 ADVISE AND COUNSEL ON FAMILY PLANNING
Counsel on the importance of family planning
Special considerations for family planning counselling during pregnancy

C17 ADVISE ON ROUTINE AND FOLLOW-UP VISITS

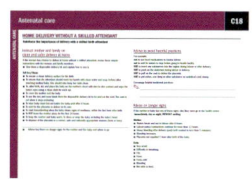

C18 HOME DELIVERY WITHOUT A SKILLED ATTENDANT
Instruct mother and family on clean and safer delivery at home
Advise to avoid harmful practices
Advise on danger signs

Assess the pregnant woman ▶ Pregnancy status, birth and emergency plan — C2

ASSESS THE PREGNANT WOMAN: PREGNANCY STATUS, BIRTH AND EMERGENCY PLAN

Use this chart to assess the pregnant woman at each of the four antenatal care visits. During first antenatal visit, prepare a birth and emergency plan using this chart and review them during following visits. Modify the birth plan if any complications arise.

ASK, CHECK RECORD	LOOK, LISTEN, FEEL	INDICATIONS	PLACE OF DELIVERY	ADVISE
ALL VISITS ■ Check duration of pregnancy. ■ Where do you plan to deliver? ■ Any vaginal bleeding since last visit? ■ Is the baby moving? (after 4 months) ■ Check record for previous complications and treatments received during this pregnancy. **FIRST VISIT** ■ How many months pregnant are you? ■ When was your last period? ■ When do you expect to deliver? ■ How old are you? ■ Have you had a baby before? If yes: ■ Check record for prior pregnancies or if there is no record ask about: → Number of prior pregnancies/deliveries → Previous miscarriage or termination → Pre-eclampsia or eclampsia in previous pregnancies → Prior caesarean section, forceps, or vacuum → Prior third degree tear → Heavy bleeding during or after delivery → Convulsions → Stillbirth or death within first 24 hours of life. → Other diseases such as diabetes, chronic hypertension, kidney, autoimmune disease → Do you use tobacco, alcohol, or any drugs?	■ Do you have any concerns? ■ Feel for trimester of pregnancy. ■ Do you use tobacco, alcohol, or any drugs? ■ Are you exposed to other people's tobacco smoke at home? → Are you exposed to other people's tobacco smoke at home? → HIV status and ARV treatment. ■ Look for caesarean scar.	■ Prior delivery by caesarean. ■ Age less than 14 years. ■ Transverse lie or other obvious malpresentation within one month of expected delivery. ■ Obvious multiple pregnancy. ■ Tubal ligation or IUD desired immediately after delivery. ■ Documented third degree tear. ■ History of or current vaginal bleeding or other complication during this pregnancy.	**REFERRAL LEVEL**	■ Explain why delivery needs to be at referral level C14. ■ Develop the birth and emergency plan C14.
		■ First birth. ■ Last baby born dead or died in first day. ■ Age less than 16 years. ■ More than six previous births. ■ Prior delivery with heavy bleeding. ■ Prior delivery with convulsions. ■ Prior delivery by forceps or vacuum. ■ HIV-infected woman.	**PRIMARY HEALTH CARE LEVEL**	■ Explain why delivery needs to be at primary health care level C14. ■ Develop the birth and emergency plan C14. ■ If yes to alcohol/tobacco/substance use; advise cessation of substance use. C10 - C13
		■ None of the above.	**ACCORDING TO WOMAN'S PREFERENCE**	■ Explain why delivery needs to be with a skilled birth attendant, preferably at a facility. ■ Develop the birth and emergency plan C14.
THIRD TRIMESTER ■ Has she been counselled on family planning? If yes, does she want tubal ligation or IUD A15.	■ Feel for obvious multiple pregnancy. ■ Feel for transverse lie. ■ Listen to fetal heart.			

 **Next:** Check for pre-eclampsia

CHECK FOR PRE-ECLAMPSIA

Screen all pregnant women at every visit.

ASK, CHECK RECORD

- Assess gestational age
- Blood pressure at the last visit?
- Eclampsia or pre-eclampsia in previous pregnancies?
- Multiple pregnancies?
- Other diseases (chronic hypertension, kidney disease or autoimmune disease)?

LOOK, LISTEN, FEEL

- Measure blood pressure in sitting position (her legs should not be dangling or crossed. Her feet should be supported or on the ground. The elbow (brachial artery) should be at the level of the heart. Ensure that the cuff is neither too wide nor too narrow).
- If diastolic blood pressure is ≥90 mmHg, repeat after 1 hour rest.
- If diastolic blood pressure is still ≥90 mmHg, ask the woman if she has:
  → severe headache
  → blurred vision
  → epigastric pain and
  → check protein in urine.

SIGNS	CLASSIFY	TREAT AND ADVISE
■ Diastolic blood pressure ≥110 mmHg and 3+ proteinuria, or ■ Diastolic blood pressure ≥90 mmHg on two readings and 2+ proteinuria, and any of: → severe headache → blurred vision → epigastric pain.	SEVERE PRE-ECLAMPSIA	■ Give magnesium sulphate **B13**. ■ Give appropriate anti-hypertensives **B14**. ■ Revise the birth plan **C2**. ■ **Refer urgently to hospital B17**.
■ Diastolic blood pressure 90-110 mmHg on two readings and 2+ proteinuria.	PRE-ECLAMPSIA	■ Revise the birth plan **C2**. ■ Refer to hospital.
■ Diastolic blood pressure ≥90 mmHg on 2 readings.	HYPERTENSION	■ Advise to reduce workload and to rest. ■ Advise on danger signs **C15**. ■ Reassess at the next antenatal visit or in 1 week if >8 months pregnant. ■ If hypertension persists after 1 week or at next visit, refer to hospital or discuss case with the doctor or midwife, if available.
■ Eclampsia or pre-eclampsia in previous pregnancies ■ Multiple pregnancy ■ Other diseases	RISK OF PRE-ECLAMPSIA	■ Give aspirin **F2**. ■ Give calcium if low dietary intake area **F2**.
■ None of the above.	NO HYPERTENSION	■ No treatment required.

Next: Check for anaemia

Assess the pregnant woman ▶ Check for pre-eclampsia

Assess the pregnant woman ▶ Check for anaemia

C4

ANTENATAL CARE

CHECK FOR ANAEMIA

Screen all pregnant women at every visit.

ASK, CHECK RECORD	LOOK, LISTEN, FEEL	SIGNS	CLASSIFY	TREAT AND ADVISE
■ Do you tire easily? ■ Are you breathless (short of breath) during routine household work? ■ Check if anti-helminthic dose was administered.	**On first visit:** ■ Measure haemoglobin **On subsequent visits:** ■ Look for conjunctival pallor. ■ Look for palmar pallor. If pallor: → Is it severe pallor? → Some pallor? → Count number of breaths in 1 minute.	■ Haemoglobin <7 g/dl. **AND/OR** ■ Severe palmar and conjunctival pallor or ■ Any pallor with any of → >30 breaths per minute → tires easily → breathlessness at rest	**SEVERE ANAEMIA**	■ Revise birth plan so as to deliver in a facility with blood transfusion services **C2**. ■ Give double dose of iron (1 tablet twice daily) for 3 months **F3**. ■ Counsel on compliance with treatment **F3**. ■ Give appropriate oral antimalarial **F4**. ■ Follow up in 2 weeks to check clinical progress, test results, and compliance with treatment. ■ **Refer urgently to hospital B17**.
		■ Haemoglobin 7-11 g/dl. ■ **OR** ■ Palmar or conjunctival pallor.	**MODERATE ANAEMIA**	■ Give double dose of iron (1 tablet twice daily) for 3 months **F3**. ■ Counsel on compliance with treatment **F3**. ■ Give appropriate oral antimalarial if not given in the past month **F4**. ■ Reassess at next antenatal visit (4-6 weeks). If anaemia persists, refer to hospital.
		■ Haemoglobin >11 g/dl. ■ No pallor.	**NO CLINICAL ANAEMIA**	■ Give iron 1 tablet once daily for 3 months **F3**. ■ Counsel on compliance with treatment **F4**.

Next: Check for syphilis

CHECK FOR SYPHILIS

Test all pregnant women at first visit. Check status at every visit.

ASK, CHECK RECORD / LOOK, LISTEN, FEEL	SIGNS	CLASSIFY	TREAT AND ADVISE
■ Have you been tested for syphilis during this pregnancy? → If not, perform the rapid plasma reagin (RPR) test **L5**. ■ If test was positive, have you and your partner been treated for syphilis? → If not, and test is positive, ask "Are you allergic to penicillin?"	■ RPR test positive.	**POSSIBLE SYPHILIS**	■ Give benzathine benzylpenicillin IM. If allergy, give erythromycin **F6**. ■ Plan to treat the newborn **K12**. ■ Encourage woman to bring her sexual partner for treatment. ■ Counsel on safer sex including use of condoms to prevent new infection **G2**.
	■ RPR test negative.	**NO SYPHILIS**	■ Counsel on safer sex including use of condoms to prevent infection **G2**.

 Next: Check for HIV status

Assess the pregnant woman ▶ Check for syphilis

Assess the pregnant woman ▶ Check for HIV status

C6

ANTENATAL CARE

CHECK FOR HIV STATUS

Test and counsel all pregnant women for HIV at the first antenatal visit. Check status at every visit.

ASK, CHECK RECORD	LOOK, LISTEN, FEEL	SIGNS	CLASSIFY	TREAT AND ADVISE
Provide key information on HIV G2. ■ What is HIV and how is HIV transmitted G2? ■ Advantage of knowing the HIV status in pregnancy G2. ■ Explain about HIV testing and counselling including confidentiality of the result G3. ■ Tell her that HIV testing will be done routinely, as other blood tests, and that she may refuse the HIV test. **Ask the woman:** ■ Have you been tested for HIV? → If not: tell her that she will be tested for HIV, unless she refuses. → If yes: Check result. (Explain to her that she has a right not to disclose the result.) → Are you taking any ARV? → Check ARV treatment plan. ■ Has the partner been tested? **Check the record** ■ When was she tested in this pregnancy? → Early (in the first trimester)? → Later?	■ Perform the Rapid HIV test if HIV-negative and not performed in this pregnancy L6.	■ Positive HIV test.	**HIV-INFECTED**	■ Give her appropriate ART G6, G9. ■ Support adherence to ART G6. ■ Counsel on implications of a positive test G3. ■ Refer her to HIV services for further assessment and initiation for lifelong ART. ■ Provide additional care for HIV-infected woman G4. ■ Provide support to the HIV-infected woman G5. ■ Counsel on benefits of disclosure (involving) and testing her partner G3. ■ Counsel on safer sex including use of condoms G2. ■ Counsel on family planning G4. ■ Counsel on infant feeding options G7. ■ Ask her to return to the next scheduled antenatal care visit.
		■ Negative HIV test.	**HIV-NEGATIVE**	■ Counsel on implications of a negative test G3. ■ Counsel on the importance of staying negative by practising safer sex, including use of condoms G2. ■ Counsel on benefits of involving and testing the partner G3. ■ Repeat HIV testing in the 3rd trimester L6.
		■ She refuses the test or is not willing to disclose the result of previous test or no test results available	**UNKNOWN HIV STATUS**	■ Assess for signs suggesting severe or advanced HIV infection C10. ■ Counsel on safer sex including use of condoms G2. ■ Counsel on benefits of involving and testing the partner G3.

▼ **Next:** Respond to observed signs or volunteered problems
If no problem, go to page C12.

RESPOND TO OBSERVED SIGNS OR VOLUNTEERED PROBLEMS

ASK, CHECK RECORD	LOOK, LISTEN, FEEL	SIGNS	CLASSIFY	TREAT AND ADVISE
IF NO FETAL MOVEMENT				
■ When did the baby last move? ■ If no movement felt, ask woman to move around for some time, reassess fetal movement.	■ Feel for fetal movements. ■ Listen for fetal heart after 6 months of pregnancy **D2**. ■ If no heart beat, repeat after 1 hour.	■ No fetal movement. ■ No fetal heart beat.	**PROBABLY DEAD BABY**	■ Inform the woman and partner about the possibility of dead baby. ■ Refer to hospital.
		■ No fetal movement but fetal heart beat present.	**WELL BABY**	■ Inform the woman that baby is fine and likely to be well but to return if problem persists.
IF RUPTURED MEMBRANES AND NO LABOUR				
■ When did the membranes rupture? ■ When is your baby due?	■ Look at pad or underwear for evidence of: → amniotic fluid → foul-smelling vaginal discharge ■ If no evidence, ask her to wear a pad. Check again in 1 hour. ■ Measure temperature.	■ Fever 38°C. ■ Foul-smelling vaginal discharge.	**UTERINE AND FETAL INFECTION**	■ Give appropriate IM/IV antibiotics **B15**. ■ **Refer urgently to hospital B17**.
		■ Rupture of membranes at <8 months of pregnancy.	**RISK OF UTERINE AND FETAL INFECTION**	■ Give corticosteroid therapy: either IM Dexamethasone or IM Betamethasone (total 24 mg in divided doses), when the following conditions are met: → gestational age is accurate: from 24 weeks and 34 weeks of gestation; → Preterm birth is considered imminent; → There is no clinical evidence of maternal infection; → Adequate childbirth care is available; → The preterm newborn can receive adequate care if needed. ■ Give Erythromycine as the antibiotic of choice **B15**. ■ **Refer urgently to hospital B17**.
		■ Rupture of membranes at >8 months of pregnancy.	**RUPTURE OF MEMBRANES**	■ Manage as Woman in childbirth **D1-D28**.

▼ **Next:** If fever or burning on urination

Respond to observed signs or volunteered problems (1)

Respond to observed signs or volunteered problems (2)

C8

ANTENATAL CARE

ASK, CHECK RECORD	LOOK, LISTEN, FEEL	SIGNS	CLASSIFY	TREAT AND ADVISE
IF FEVER OR BURNING ON URINATION				
■ Have you had fever? ■ Do you have burning on urination?	■ If history of fever or feels hot: → Measure axillary temperature. → Look or feel for stiff neck. → Look for lethargy. ■ Percuss flanks for tenderness.	■ Fever >38°C and any of: → very fast breathing or → stiff neck → lethargy → very weak/not able to stand.	**VERY SEVERE FEBRILE DISEASE**	■ Insert IV line and give fluids slowly **B9**. ■ Give appropriate IM/IV antibiotics **B15**. ■ Give appropriate antimalarial IV/IM (if malaria is confirmed) **B16**. ■ Give glucose **B16**. ■ **Refer urgently to hospital B17**.
		■ Fever >38°C and any of: → Flank pain → Burning on urination.	**UPPER URINARY TRACT INFECTION**	■ Give appropriate IM/IV antibiotics **B15**. ■ **Refer urgently to hospital B17**.
		■ Fever >38°C or history of fever (in last 48 hours).	**MALARIA**	■ Confirm malaria with parasitological diagnosis ■ Give appropriate oral antimalarial **F4**. ■ If no improvement in 2 days or condition is worse, refer to hospital.
		■ Burning on urination.	**LOWER URINARY TRACT INFECTION**	■ Give appropriate oral antibiotics **F5**. ■ Encourage her to drink more fluids. ■ If no improvement in 2 days or condition is worse, refer to hospital.

Next: If vaginal discharge

ASK, CHECK RECORD	LOOK, LISTEN, FEEL	SIGNS	CLASSIFY	TREAT AND ADVISE
IF VAGINAL DISCHARGE				
■ Have you noticed changes in your vaginal discharge? ■ Do you have itching at the vulva? ■ Has your partner had a urinary problem? If partner is present in the clinic, ask the woman if she feels comfortable if you ask him similar questions. ■ If yes, ask him if he has: ■ urethral discharge or pus. ■ burning on passing urine. If partner could not be approached, explain importance of partner assessment and treatment to avoid reinfection. Schedule follow-up appointment for woman and partner (if possible).	■ Separate the labia and look for abnormal vaginal discharge: → amount → colour → odour/smell. ■ If no discharge is seen, examine with a gloved finger and look at the discharge on the glove.	■ Abnormal vaginal discharge. ■ Partner has urethral discharge or burning on passing urine.	**POSSIBLE GONORRHOEA OR CHLAMYDIA INFECTION**	■ Give appropriate oral antibiotics to woman F5. ■ Treat partner with appropriate oral antibiotics F5. ■ Counsel on safer sex including use of condoms G2.
		■ Curd like vaginal discharge. ■ Intense vulval itching.	**POSSIBLE CANDIDA INFECTION**	■ Give clotrimazole F5. ■ Counsel on safer sex including use of condoms G2.
		■ Abnormal vaginal discharge	**POSSIBLE BACTERIAL OR TRICHOMONAS INFECTION**	■ Give metronidazole to woman F5. ■ Counsel on safer sex including use of condoms G2.

▼ **Next:** If signs suggesting HIV infection

Respond to observed signs or volunteered problems (3)

Respond to observed signs or volunteered problems (4) — C10

ANTENATAL CARE

| ASK, CHECK RECORD | LOOK, LISTEN, FEEL | SIGNS | CLASSIFY | TREAT AND ADVISE |

IF SIGNS SUGGESTING SEVERE OR ADVANCED HIV INFECTION

(HIV status unknown and refused HIV testing)

- Have you lost weight?
- Have you got diarrhoea (continuous or intermittent)?
  How long, >1 month?
- Do you have fever?
  How long (>1 month)?
- Have you had cough?
  How long >1 month?
- Have you any difficulty in breathing?
  How long (more than >1 month)?
- Have you noticed any change in vaginal discharge?

Assess if in high risk group:
- Occupational exposure?
- Multiple sexual partners?
- Intravenous drug use?

- Look for visible wasting.
- Look at the skin:
  → Is there a rash?
  → Are there blisters along the ribs on one side of the body?
- Feel the head, neck and underarm for enlarged lymph nodes.
- Look for ulcers and white patches in the mouth (thrush).
- Look for any abnormal vaginal discharge **C9**.

- History of blood transfusion?
- Illness or death from AIDS in a sexual partners?
- History of forced sex?

- Two of these signs:
  → weight loss or no weight gain visible wasting
  → diarrhoea >1 month
  → cough more than 1 month or difficulty breathing
  → itching rash
  → blisters along the ribs on one side of the body
  → enlarged lymph nodes
  → cracks/ulcers around lips/mouth
  → abnormal vaginal discharge.
OR
- One of the above signs and
  → one or more other signs or
  → from a risk group.

STRONG LIKELIHOOD OF SEVERE OR ADVANCED SYMPTOMATIC HIV INFECTION

- Refer to clinic or hospital where advanced treatment services are offered based on severity.

IF SMOKING USING TOBACCO, ALCOHOL OR DRUG ABUSE, OR HISTORY OF VIOLENCE

Assess if dependent on:
- Tobacco use?
- Alcohol?
- drug use?

- Counsel on stopping use of tobacco and avoiding exposure to second-hand smoke
- For alcohol/drug abuse, refer to specialized care providers.
- For counselling on violence, see **H4**.

Next: If cough or breathing difficulty

ASK, CHECK RECORD	LOOK, LISTEN, FEEL	SIGNS	CLASSIFY	TREAT AND ADVISE
IF COUGH OR BREATHING DIFFICULTY				
■ How long have you been coughing? ■ How long have you had difficulty in breathing? ■ Do you have chest pain? ■ Do you have any blood in sputum? ■ Do you smoke tobacco? ■ Are you exposed to other people's smoke at home?	■ Look for breathlessness. ■ Listen for wheezing. ■ Measure temperature.	■ At least 2 of the following signs: ■ Fever >38°C. ■ Breathlessness. ■ Chest pain.	POSSIBLE PNEUMONIA	■ Give first dose of appropriate IM/IV antibiotics B15. ■ **Refer urgently to hospital** B17.
		■ At least 1 of the following signs: ■ Cough or breathing difficulty for >3 weeks ■ Blood in sputum ■ Wheezing	POSSIBLE CHRONIC LUNG DISEASE	■ Refer to hospital for assessment. ■ If severe wheezing, refer urgently to hospital.
		■ Fever <38°C, and ■ Cough <3 weeks.	UPPER RESPIRATORY TRACT INFECTION	■ Advise safe, soothing remedy. ■ If smoking, counsel to stop smoking ■ Avoid exposure to second-hand smoke
IF TAKING ANTI-TUBERCULOSIS DRUGS				
■ Are you taking anti-tuberculosis (TB) drugs? If yes, since when? ■ Does the treatment include injection (streptomycin)?		■ Taking anti-tuberculosis drugs. ■ Receiving injectable anti-tuberculosis drugs.	TUBERCULOSIS	■ If anti-tubercular treatment includes streptomycin (injection), refer the woman to district hospital for revision of treatment as streptomycin is ototoxic to the fetus. ■ If treatment does not include streptomycin, assure the woman that the drugs are not harmful to her baby, and urge her to continue treatment for a successful outcome of pregnancy. ■ If her sputum is TB positive within 2 months of delivery, plan to give INH prophylaxis to the newborn K13. ■ Offer HIV testing and counselling G2-G3. ■ If smoking, counsel to stop smoking, and avoid exposure to second-hand smoke ■ Advise to screen immediate family members and close contacts for tuberculosis.

 Next: Give preventive measures

Respond to observed signs or volunteered problems (5)

Give preventive measures

C12

GIVE PREVENTIVE MEASURES

Advise and counsel all pregnant women at every antenatal care visit.

ASK, CHECK RECORD	TREAT AND ADVISE
■ Check tetanus toxoid (TT) immunization status.	■ Give tetanus toxoid if due **F2**. ■ If TT1, plan to give TT2 at next visit.
■ Check woman's supply of the prescribed dose of iron/folate and aspirin, calcium and ART if prescribed.	■ Give 3 month's supply of iron, aspirin, calcium and ART if prescribed and counsel on adherence and safety of each medicine **F2**, **F3**, **G6**, **G9**.
■ Check when last dose of mebendazole given.	■ Give mebendazole once in second or third trimester **F3**.
■ Check when last dose of an antimalarial given. ■ Ask if she (and children) are sleeping under insecticide treated bednets.	■ Give intermittent preventive treatment in second and third trimesters **F4**. ■ Encourage sleeping under insecticide treated bednets.
	First visit ■ Develop a birth and emergency plan **C14**. ■ Counsel on nutrition **C13**. ■ Counsel on importance of exclusive breastfeeding **K2**. ■ Counsel on stopping use of tobacco and alcohol and drug abuse; and to avoid second-hand smoke exposure. ■ Counsel on safer sex including use of condoms. **All visits** ■ Review and update the birth and emergency plan according to new findings **C14-C15**. ■ Advise on when to seek care: **C17** → routine visits → follow-up visits → danger signs → HIV-related visits. **Third trimester** ■ Counsel on family planning **C16**. ■ Ask and counsel on abstinence from use of tobacco, alcohol and drugs, and to avoid second-hand smoke exposure.
■ Record all visits and treatments given.	

Next: If cough or breathing difficulty

ADVISE AND COUNSEL ON NUTRITION AND SELF-CARE AND SUBSTANCE ABUSE

Use the information and counselling sheet to support your interaction with the woman, her partner and family.

Counsel on nutrition

- Advise the woman to eat a greater amount and variety of healthy foods, such as meat, fish, oils, nuts, seeds, cereals, beans, vegetables, cheese, milk, to help her feel well and strong (give examples of types of food and how much to eat).
- Spend more time on nutrition counselling with very thin, adolescent and HIV-infected woman.
- Determine if there are important taboos about foods which are nutritionally important for good health. Advise the woman against these taboos.
- Talk to family members such as the partner and mother-in-law, to encourage them to help ensure the woman eats enough and avoids hard physical work.

Advise on self-care during pregnancy

Advise the woman to:
- Take iron tablets **F3**.
- Rest and avoid lifting heavy objects.
- Sleep under an insecticide impregnated bednet.
- Counsel on safer sex including use of condoms, if at risk for STI or HIV **G2**.
- Avoid alcohol and smoking during pregnancy.
- NOT to take medication unless prescribed at the health centre/hospital.

Counsel on Substance Abuse:
- Avoid tobacco use during pregnancy.
- Avoid exposure to second-hand smoke.
- Do not take any drugs or Nicotine Replacement Therapy for tobacco cessation.

Counsel on alcohol use:
- Avoid alcohol during pregnancy.

Counsel on drug use:
- Avoid use of drugs during pregnancy.

Develop a birth and emergency plan (1)　　C14

DEVELOP A BIRTH AND EMERGENCY PLAN

Use the information and counselling sheet to support your interaction with the woman, her partner and family.

Facility delivery

Explain why birth in a facility is recommended
- Any complication can develop during delivery - they are not always predictable.
- A facility has staff, equipment, supplies and drugs available to provide best care if needed, and a referral system.
- If HIV-infected she will need appropriate ARV treatment for herself and her baby during childbirth.
- Complications are more common in HIV-infected women and their newborns. HIV-infected women should deliver in a facility.

Advise how to prepare
Review the arrangements for delivery:
- How will she get there? Will she have to pay for transport?
- How much will it cost to deliver at the facility? How will she pay?
- Can she start saving straight away?
- Who will go with her for support during labour and delivery?
- Who will help while she is away to care for her home and other children?

Advise when to go
- If the woman lives near the facility, she should go at the first signs of labour.
- If living far from the facility, she should go 2-3 weeks before baby due date and stay either at the maternity waiting home or with family or friends near the facility.
- Advise to ask for help from the community, if needed **I2**.

Advise what to bring
- Home-based maternal record.
- Clean cloths for washing, drying and wrapping the baby.
- Additional clean cloths to use as sanitary pads after birth.
- Clothes for mother and baby.
- Food and water for woman and support person.

Home delivery with a skilled attendant

Advise how to prepare
- Review the following with her:
- Who will be the companion during labour and delivery?
- Who will be close by for at least 24 hours after delivery?
- Who will help to care for her home and other children?
- Advise to call the skilled attendant at the first signs of labour.
- Advise to have her home-based maternal record ready.
- Advise to ask for help from the community, if needed **I2**.

Explain supplies needed for home delivery
- Warm spot for the birth with a clean surface or a clean cloth.
- Clean cloths of different sizes: for the bed, for drying and wrapping the baby, for cleaning the baby's eyes, for the birth attendant to wash and dry her hands, for use as sanitary pads.
- Blankets.
- Buckets of clean water and some way to heat this water.
- Soap.
- Bowls: 2 for washing and 1 for the placenta.
- Plastic for wrapping the placenta.

ANTENATAL CARE

Advise on labour signs

Advise to go to the facility or contact the skilled birth attendant if any of the following signs:

- a bloody sticky discharge.
- painful contractions every 20 minutes or less.
- waters have broken.

Advise on danger signs

Advise to go to the hospital/health centre **immediately, day or night, WITHOUT waiting** if any of the following signs:

- vaginal bleeding.
- convulsions.
- severe headaches with blurred vision.
- fever and too weak to get out of bed.
- severe abdominal pain.
- fast or difficult breathing.

- She should go to the health centre **as soon as possible** if any of the following signs:
- fever.
- abdominal pain.
- feels ill.
- swelling of fingers, face, legs.

Discuss how to prepare for an emergency in pregnancy

- Discuss emergency issues with the woman and her partner/family:
  → where will she go?
  → how will they get there?
  → how much it will cost for services and transport?
  → can she start saving straight away?
  → who will go with her for support during labour and delivery?
  → who will care for her home and other children?
- Advise the woman to ask for help from the community, if needed I1-I3.
- Advise her to bring her home-based maternal record to the health centre, even for an emergency visit.

ANTENATAL CARE

Develop a birth and emergency plan (2)

C15

Advise and counsel on family planning C16

ADVISE AND COUNSEL ON FAMILY PLANNING

Counsel on the importance of family planning

- If appropriate, ask the woman if she would like her partner or another family member to be included in the counselling session.
- Explain that after birth, if she has sex and is not exclusively breastfeeding, she can become pregnant as soon as four weeks after delivery. Therefore it is important to start thinking early on about what family planning method they will use.
    - → Ask about plans for having more children. If she (and her partner) want more children, advise that waiting at least 2 years before trying to become pregnant again is good for the mother and for the baby's health.
    - → Information on when to start a method after delivery will vary depending whether a woman is breastfeeding or not.
    - → Make arrangements for the woman to see a family planning counsellor, or counsel her directly (see the Decision-making tool for family planning providers and clients for information on methods and on the counselling process).
- Counsel on safer sex including use of condoms for dual protection from sexually transmitted infections (STI) or HIV and pregnancy. Promote especially if at risk for STI or HIV G4.
- For HIV-infected women, see G4 for family planning considerations
- Her partner can decide to have a vasectomy (male sterilization) at any time.

Method options for the non-breastfeeding woman

Can be used immediately postpartum	Condoms Progestogen-only oral contraceptives Progestogen-only injectables Implant Spermicide Female sterilization (within 7 days or delay 6 weeks) Copper IUD or levonorgestrel-releasing intrauterine device (LNG-IUD) (immediately following expulsion of placenta or within 48 hours)
Delay 3 weeks	Combined oral contraceptives Combined injectables Diaphragm Fertility awareness methods

Special considerations for family planning counselling during pregnancy

Counselling should be given during the third trimester of pregnancy.

- If the woman chooses female sterilization:
    - → can be performed immediately postpartum if no sign of infection (ideally within 7 days, or delay for 6 weeks).
    - → plan for delivery in hospital or health centre where they are trained to carry out the procedure.
    - → ensure counselling and informed consent prior to labour and delivery.
- If the woman chooses an intrauterine device (IUD):
    - → can be inserted immediately postpartum if no sign of infection (up to 48 hours, or delay 4 weeks)
    - → plan for delivery in hospital or health centre where they are trained to insert the IUD.

Method options for the breastfeeding woman

Can be used immediately postpartum	Lactational amenorrhoea method (LAM) Condoms Spermicide Female sterilization (within 7 days or delay 6 weeks) Copper IUD or levonorgestrel-releasing intrauterine device (LNG-IUD) (within 48 hours or delay 4 weeks)
6 weeks postpartum	Breastfeeding women who are < 6 weeks postpartum can generally use progestogen-only pills (POPs) and levonorgestrel (LNG) and etonogestrel (ETG) implants. Breastfeeding women who are < 6 weeks postpartum generally should not use progestogen-only injectables (POIs) (Depot medroxyprogesterone acetate – DMPA or Norethisterone enanthate - NET-EN).
6 weeks to < 6 months	Breastfeeding women who are >= 6 weeks to < 6 months postpartum can generally use progestogen-only pills (POPs), POIs and levonorgestrel (LNG) and etonogestrel (ETG) implants.
6 months	Breastfeeding women who are >= 6 weeks to < 6 months postpartum can generally use progestogen-only pills (POPs), POIs and levonorgestrel (LNG) and etonogestrel (ETG) implants.

ADVISE ON ROUTINE AND FOLLOW-UP VISITS

Encourage the woman to bring her partner or family member to at least 1 visit.

Routine antenatal care visits

1st visit	Before 4 months	Before 16 weeks
2nd visit	6 months	24-28 weeks
3rd visit	8 months	30-32 weeks
4th visit	9 months	36-38 weeks

- All pregnant women should have 4 routine antenatal visits.
- First antenatal contact should be as early in pregnancy as possible.
- During the last visit, inform the woman to return if she does not deliver within 2 weeks after the expected date of delivery.
- More frequent visits or different schedules may be required according to national malaria or HIV policies.
- If women is HIV-infected ensure a visit between 26-28 weeks.

Follow-up visits

If the problem was:	Return in:
Hypertension	1 week if >8 months pregnant
Severe anaemia	2 weeks
HIV-infection	2 weeks after HIV testing

Advise on routine and follow-up visits

Antenatal care

C18

HOME DELIVERY WITHOUT A SKILLED ATTENDANT

Reinforce the importance of delivery with a skilled birth attendant

Instruct mother and family on clean and safer delivery at home

If the woman has chosen to deliver at home without a skilled attendant, review these simple instructions with the woman and family members.
- Give them a disposable delivery kit and explain how to use it.

Tell her/them:
- To ensure a clean delivery surface for the birth.
- To ensure that the attendant should wash her hands with clean water and soap before/after touching mother/baby. She should also keep her nails clean.
- To, after birth, dry and place the baby on the mother's chest with skin-to-skin contact and wipe the baby's eyes using a clean cloth for each eye.
- To cover the mother and the baby.
- To use the ties and razor blade from the disposable delivery kit to tie and cut the cord. The cord is cut when it stops pulsating.
- To wipe baby clean but not bathe the baby until after 24 hours (if this is not possible due to cultural reasons, bathing should be delayed for at least six hours).
- To wait for the placenta to deliver on its own.
- To start breastfeeding when the baby shows signs of readiness, within the first hour after birth.
- To NOT leave the mother alone for the first 24 hours.
- To keep the mother and baby warm. To dress or wrap the baby, including the baby's head.
- To dispose of the placenta in a correct, safe and culturally appropriate manner (burn or bury).
- Apply 7.1% chlorhexidine digluconate (gel or liquid) to the umbilical cord stump once daily for the first week of life. In areas where chlorhexidine is not used for umbilical cord care keep cord clean and dry.

- Advise her/them on danger signs for the mother and the baby and where to go.

Advise to avoid harmful practices

For example:
NOT to use local medications to hasten labour.
NOT to wait for waters to stop before going to health facility.
NOT to insert any substances into the vagina during labour or after delivery.
NOT to push on the abdomen during labour or delivery.
NOT to pull on the cord to deliver the placenta.
NOT to put any substance on umbilical cord/stump other than 7.1% chlorhexidine digluconate (where recommended by health authority).

Encourage helpful traditional practices:

 _____

_____

Advise on danger signs

If the mother or baby has any of these signs, she/they must go to the health centre **immediately, day or night, WITHOUT waiting**

Mother
- Waters break and not in labour after 6 hours.
- Labour pains/contractions continue for more than 12 hours.
- Heavy bleeding after delivery (pad/cloth soaked in less than 5 minutes).
- Bleeding increases.
- Placenta not expelled 1 hour after birth of the baby.

Baby
- Very small.
- Difficulty in breathing.
- Fits.
- Fever.
- Feels cold.
- Bleeding.
- Not able to feed

Childbirth: labour, delivery and immediate postpartum care

CHILDBIRTH: LABOUR, DELIVERY AND IMMEDIATE POSTPARTUM CARE

D2 EXAMINE THE WOMAN IN LABOUR OR WITH RUPTURED MEMBRES

D3 DECIDE STAGE OF LABOUR

D4 RESPOND TO OBSTETRICAL PROBLEMS ON ADMISSION (1)

D5 RESPOND TO OBSTETRICAL PROBLEMS ON ADMISSION (2)

D6 GIVE SUPPORTIVE CARE THROUGHOUT LABOUR

D7 BIRTH COMPANION

D8 FIRST STAGE OF LABOUR (1): WHEN THE WOMAN IS NOT IN ACTIVE LABOUR

D9 FIRST STAGE OF LABOUR (2): IN ACTIVE LABOUR

D10 SECOND STAGE OF LABOUR: DELIVER THE BABY AND GIVE IMMEDIATE NEWBORN CARE (1)

D11 SECOND STAGE OF LABOUR: DELIVER THE BABY AND GIVE IMMEDIATE NEWBORN CARE (2)

D12 THIRD STAGE OF LABOUR: DELIVER THE PLACENTA (1)

D13 THIRD STAGE OF LABOUR: DELIVER THE PLACENTA (2)

D14 RESPOND TO PROBLEMS DURING LABOUR AND DELIVERY (1)
If fetal heart rate <120 or >160bpm

D15 RESPOND TO PROBLEMS DURING LABOUR AND DELIVERY (2)
If prolapsed cord

D16 RESPOND TO PROBLEMS DURING LABOUR AND DELIVERY (3)
If breech presentation

D17 RESPOND TO PROBLEMS DURING LABOUR AND DELIVERY (4)
If stuck shoulders

D18 RESPOND TO PROBLEMS DURING LABOUR AND DELIVERY (5)
If multiple births

D19 CARE OF THE MOTHER AND NEWBORN WITHIN FIRST HOUR OF DELIVERY OF PLACENTA

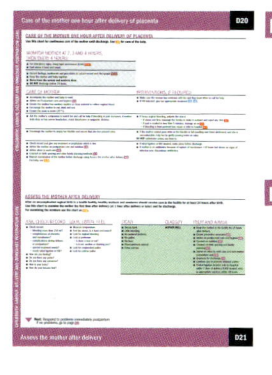

D20 CARE OF THE MOTHER ONE HOUR AFTER DELIVERY OF PLACENTA

D21 ASSESS THE MOTHER AFTER DELIVERY

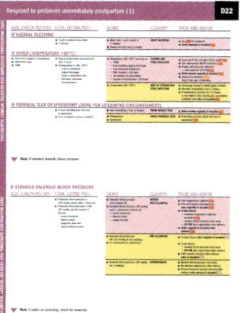

D22 RESPOND TO PROBLEMS IMMEDIATELY POSTPARTUM (1)
If vaginal bleeding
If fever
If perineal tear or episiotomy

D23 RESPOND TO PROBLEMS IMMEDIATELY POSTPARTUM (2)
If elevated diastolic blood pressure

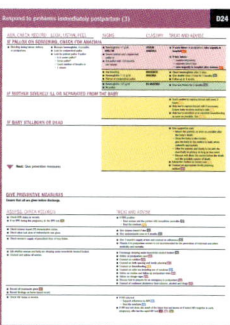

D24 RESPOND TO PROBLEMS IMMEDIATELY POSTPARTUM (3)
If pallor on screening, check for anaemia
If mother severely ill or separated from baby
If baby stillborn or dead

D25 GIVE PREVENTIVE MEASURES

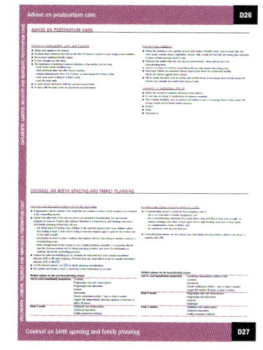

D26 ADVISE ON POSTPARTUM CARE
Advise on postpartum care and hygiene
Counsel on nutrition

D27 COUNSEL ON BIRTH SPACING AND FAMILY PLANNING
Counsel on importance of family planning
Lactation and amenorrhoea method (LAM)

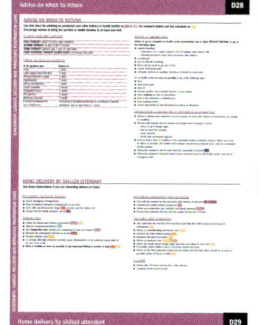

D28 ADVISE ON WHEN TO RETURN
Routine postpartum visits
Advise on danger signs
Discuss how to prepare for an emergency postpartum

D29 HOME DELIVERY BY SKILLED ATTENDANT
Preparation for home delivery
Delivery care
Immediate postpartum care of the mother
Postpartum care of the newborn

- Always begin with **Rapid assessment and management (RAM)** `B3-B7`.

- Next, use the chart on **Examine the woman in labour or with ruptured membranes** `D2-D3` to assess the clinical situation and obstetrical history, and decide the stage of labour.

- If an abnormal sign is identified, use the charts on **Respond to obstetrical problems** on admission `D4-D5`.

- Care for the woman according to the stage of labour `D8-D13` and respond to problems during labour and delivery as on `D14-D18`.

- Use **Give supportive care throughout labour** `D6-D7` to provide support and care throughout labour and delivery.

- Record findings continually on labour record and partograph `N4-N6`.

- Keep mother and baby in labour room for one hour after delivery and use charts **Care of the mother and newborn within first hour of delivery placenta** on `D19`.

- Next use **Care of the mother after the first hour following delivery of placenta** `D20` to provide care until discharge. Use chart on `D25` to provide **Preventive measures** and **Advise on postpartum care** `D26-D28` to advise on care, danger signs, when to seek routine or emergency care, and family planning.

- Examine the mother for discharge using chart on `D21`.

- **Do not** discharge mother from the facility before 24 hours after birth.

- If the mother is HIV-infected or adolescent, or has special needs, see `G1-G11` `H1-H4`.

- If attending a delivery at the woman's home, see `D29`.

Childbirth: labour, delivery and immediate postpartum care

Examine the woman in labour or with ruptured membranes — D2

CHILDBIRTH: LABOUR, DELIVERY AND IMMEDIATE POSTPARTUM CARE

EXAMINE THE WOMAN IN LABOUR OR WITH RUPTURED MEMBRANES

First do Rapid assessment and management `B3-B7`. Then use this chart to assess the woman's and fetal status and decide stage of labour.

ASK, CHECK RECORD

History of this labour:
- When did contractions begin?
- How frequent are contractions? How strong?
- Have your waters broken? If yes, when? Were they clear or green?
- Have you had any bleeding? If yes, when? How much?
- Is the baby moving?
- Do you have any concern?

Check record, or if no record:
- Ask when the delivery is expected.
- Determine if preterm (less than 37 weeks of gestation).
- Review the birth plan.

If prior pregnancies:
- Number of prior pregnancies/deliveries.
- Any prior caesarean section, forceps, or vacuum, or other complication such as postpartum haemorrhage?
- Any prior third or fourth degree tears?

Current pregnancy:
- RPR status `C5`.
- Hb results `C4`.
- Tetanus immunization status `F2`.
- HIV status `C6`.
- Infant feeding plan `G7-G8`.
- Receiving any medicine.

LOOK, LISTEN, FEEL

- Observe the woman's response to contractions:
  → Is she coping well or is she distressed?
- Is she pushing or grunting?
- Check abdomen for:
  → caesarean section scar.
  → horizontal ridge across lower abdomen (if present, empty bladder `B12` and observe again).
- Feel abdomen for:
  → contractions frequency, duration, any continuous contractions?
  → fetal lie—longitudinal or transverse?
  → fetal presentation—head, breech, other?
  → more than one fetus?
  → fetal movement.
- Listen to the fetal heart beat:
  → Count number of beats in 1 minute.
  → If less than 100 beats per minute, or more than 180, turn woman on her left side and count again.
- Measure blood pressure.
- Measure temperature.
- Look for pallor.
- Look for sunken eyes, dry mouth.
- Pinch the skin of the forearm: does it go back quickly?

Next: Perform vaginal examination and decide stage of labour.

DECIDE STAGE OF LABOUR

ASK, CHECK RECORD

- Explain to the woman that you will give her a vaginal examination and ask for her consent.

LOOK, LISTEN, FEEL

- Look at vulva for:
  → bulging perineum
  → any visible fetal parts
  → vaginal bleeding
  → leaking amniotic fluid; if yes, is it meconium stained, foul-smelling?
  → warts, keloid tissue or scars that may interfere with delivery.
  → Check uterine contractions

Perform vaginal examination
- **DO NOT** shave the perineal area.
- Prepare:
  → sterile gloves
  → swabs, pads.
- Wash hands with soap before and after each examination.
- Wash vulva and perineal areas with tap water.
- Put on sterile gloves.
- Position the woman with legs flexed and apart.

DO NOT perform vaginal examination if bleeding now or at any time after 7 months of pregnancy.

- Perform gentle vaginal examination (do not start during a contraction):
  → Determine cervical dilatation in centimetres.
  → Feel for presenting part. Is it hard, round and smooth (the head)? If not, identify the presenting part.
  → Feel for membranes – are they intact?
  → Feel for cord – is it felt? Is it pulsating? If so, act immediately as on **D15**.

SIGNS | CLASSIFY | MANAGE

SIGNS	CLASSIFY	MANAGE
■ Bulging thin perineum, vagina gaping and head visible, full cervical dilatation.	**IMMINENT DELIVERY**	■ See second stage of labour **D10-D11**. ■ Record in partograph **N5**.
■ Cervical dilatation: → multigravida ≥5 cm → primigravida ≥6 cm	**LATE ACTIVE LABOUR**	■ See first stage of labour – active labour **D9**. ■ Start plotting partograph **N5**. ■ Record in labour record **N5**.
■ Cervical dilatation ≥4 cm.	**EARLY ACTIVE LABOUR**	
■ Cervical dilatation: 0-3 cm; contractions weak and <2 in 10 minutes.	**NOT YET IN ACTIVE LABOUR**	■ See first stage of labour – not active labour **D8**. ■ Record in labour record **N4**.

 Next: Respond to obstetrical problems on admission.

Decide stage of labour

Respond to obstetrical problems on admission — D4

RESPOND TO OBSTETRICAL PROBLEMS ON ADMISSION

Use this chart if abnormal findings on assessing pregnancy and fetal status D2-D3.

SIGNS	CLASSIFY	TREAT AND ADVISE
■ Transverse lie. ■ Continuous contractions. ■ Constant pain between contractions. ■ Sudden and severe abdominal pain. ■ Horizontal ridge across lower abdomen. ■ Labour >24 hours (with no progress in dilatation or fetal descent).	OBSTRUCTED LABOUR	■ If distressed, insert an IV line and give fluids B9. ■ If in labour >24 hours. ■ **Refer urgently to hospital** B17.

FOR ALL SITUATIONS IN RED BELOW, **REFER URGENTLY TO HOSPITAL IF IN EARLY LABOUR,** MANAGE ONLY IF IN LATE LABOUR

SIGNS	CLASSIFY	TREAT AND ADVISE
■ Rupture of membranes and any of: → Fever >38°C → Foul-smelling vaginal discharge.	UTERINE AND FETAL INFECTION	■ Give appropriate IM/IV antibiotics B15. ■ If late labour, deliver and refer to hospital after delivery B17. ■ Plan to treat newborn J5.
■ Rupture of membranes at <8 months of pregnancy.	RISK OF UTERINE AND FETAL INFECTION AND RESPIRATORY DISTRESS SYNDROME	■ Give appropriate IM/IV antibiotics B15. ■ If late labour, deliver D10-D28. ■ Discontinue antibiotic for mother after delivery if no signs of infection. ■ Plan to treat newborn J5.
■ Diastolic blood pressure >90 mmHg.	PRE-ECLAMPSIA	■ Assess further and manage as on D23.
■ Severe palmar and conjunctival pallor and/or haemoglobin <7 g/dl.	SEVERE ANAEMIA	■ Manage as on D24.
■ Breech or other malpresentation D16. ■ Multiple pregnancy D18. ■ Fetal distress D14. ■ Prolapsed cord D15.	OBSTETRICAL COMPLICATION	■ Follow specific instructions (see page numbers in left column).

CHILDBIRTH: LABOUR, DELIVERY AND IMMEDIATE POSTPARTUM CARE

SIGNS	CLASSIFY	TREAT AND ADVISE
■ Warts, keloid tissue that appear in perineum to interfere with delivery. ■ Prior third degree tear. ■ Bleeding any time in third trimester. ■ Prior delivery by: → caesarean section → forceps or vacuum delivery. ■ Age less than 14 years.	RISK OF OBSTETRICAL COMPLICATION	■ DO NOT routinely perform episiotomy. ■ In the presence of physical obstruction due lesions or scar tissue in the perineum, a decision to perform episiotomy may be taken D10-D11. ■ If late labour, deliver D10-D28. ■ Have help available during delivery.
■ Labour before 8 completed months of pregnancy (more than one month before estimated date of delivery).	PRETERM LABOUR	■ Reassess fetal presentation (breech more common). ■ If woman is lying, encourage her to lie on her left side. ■ Call for help during delivery. ■ Routine delivery by caesarean section for the purpose of improving preterm newborn outcomes is not recommended, regardless of cephalic or breech presentation. ■ The use of magnesium sulfate is recommended for women at risk of imminent preterm birth before 32 weeks of gestation for prevention of cerebral palsy in the infant and child B13. ■ Conduct delivery very carefully as small baby may pop out suddenly. In particular, control delivery of the head. ■ Prepare equipment for resuscitation of newborn K11.
■ Fetal heart rate <120 or >160 beats per minute.	POSSIBLE FETAL DISTRESS	■ Manage as on D14.
■ Rupture of membranes at term and before labour.	RUPTURE OF MEMBRANES	■ Routine antibiotic administration is not recommended for women with prelabour rupture of membranes at (near) term B15. ■ Plan to treat the newborn J3-J5.
■ If two or more of the following signs: → thirsty → sunken eyes → dry mouth → skin pinch goes back slowly.	DEHYDRATION	■ Give oral fluids. ■ If not able to drink, give 1 litre IV fluids over 3 hours B9.
■ HIV test positive. ■ Taking ARV treatment or prophylaxis.	HIV-INFECTED	■ Ensure that the woman takes ARV drugs as prescribed G6, G9. ■ Support her choice of infant feeding G7-G8.
■ No fetal movement, and ■ No fetal heart beat on repeated examination	POSSIBLE FETAL DEATH	■ Explain to the parents that the baby is not doing well.

▼ **Next:** Give supportive care throughout labour

Respond to obstetrical problems on admission

D5

Give supportive care throughout labour D6

GIVE SUPPORTIVE CARE THROUGHOUT LABOUR

Use this chart to provide a supportive, encouraging atmosphere for birth, respectful of the woman's wishes.

Communication
- Explain all procedures, seek permission, and discuss findings with the woman.
- Keep her informed about the progress of labour.
- Praise her, encourage and reassure her that things are going well.
- Ensure and respect privacy during examinations and discussions.
- If known HIV-infected, find out what she has told the companion. Respect her wishes.

Cleanliness
- Encourage the woman to bathe or shower or wash herself and genitals at the onset of labour.
- Wash the vulva and perineal areas before each examination.
- Wash your hands with soap before and after each examination. Use sterile gloves for vaginal examination.
- Ensure cleanliness of labour and birthing area(s).
- Clean up spills immediately.
- **DO NOT** give enema.

Mobility
- Encourage the woman to walk around freely during the first stage of labour.
- Support the woman's choice of position (left lateral, squating, kneeling, standing supported by the companion) for each stage of labour and delivery.

Urination
- Encourage the woman to empty her bladder frequently. Remind her every 2 hours.

Eating, drinking
- Encourage the woman to eat and drink as she wishes throughout labour.
- Nutritious liquid drinks are important, even in late labour.
- If the woman has visible severe wasting or tires during labour, make sure she eats and drinks.

Breathing technique
- Teach her to notice her normal breathing.
- Encourage her to breathe out more slowly, making a sighing noise, and to relax with each breath.
- If she feels dizzy, unwell, is feeling pins-and-needles (tingling) in her face, hands and feet, encourage her to breathe more slowly.
- To prevent pushing at the end of first stage of labour, teach her to pant, to breathe with an open mouth, to take in 2 short breaths followed by a long breath out.
- During delivery of the head, ask her not to push but to breathe steadily or to pant.

Pain and discomfort relief
- Suggest change of position.
- Encourage mobility, as comfortable for her.
- Encourage companion to:
  → massage the woman's back if she finds this helpful.
  → hold the woman's hand and sponge her face between contractions.
- Encourage her to use the breathing technique.
- Encourage warm bath or shower, if available.

- **If woman is distressed or anxious, investigate the cause** D2-D3.
- **If pain is constant (persisting between contractions) and very severe or sudden in onset** D4.

Birth companion

- Encourage support from the chosen birth companion throughout labour.
- Describe to the birth companion what she or he should do:
  - → Always be with the woman.
  - → Encourage her.
  - → Help her to breathe and relax.
  - → Rub her back, wipe her brow with a wet cloth, do other supportive actions.
  - → Give support using local practices which do not disturb labour or delivery.
  - → Encourage woman to move around freely as she wishes and to adopt the position of her choice.
  - → Encourage her to drink fluids and eat as she wishes.
  - → Assist her to the toilet when needed.

- Ask the birth companion to call for help if:
  - → The woman is bearing down with contractions.
  - → There is vaginal bleeding.
  - → She is suddenly in much more pain.
  - → She loses consciousness or has fits.
  - → There is any other concern.

- Tell the birth companion what she or he **should NOT do** and explain why:
- **DO NOT** encourage woman to push.
- **DO NOT** give advice other than that given by the health worker.
- **DO NOT** keep woman in bed if she wants to move around.

Birth companion

D7

First stage of labour (1): when the woman is not in active labour

D8

FIRST STAGE OF LABOUR: NOT IN ACTIVE LABOUR

Use this chart for care of the woman when NOT IN ACTIVE LABOUR, when cervix dilated 0-3 cm and contractions are weak, less than 2 in 10 minutes.

MONITOR EVERY HOUR:

- For emergency signs, using rapid assessment (RAM) **B3-B7**.
- Frequency, intensity and duration of contractions.
- Fetal heart rate **D14**.
- Mood and behaviour (distressed, anxious) **D6**.

- Record findings regularly in Labour record and Partograph **N4-N6**.
- Record time of rupture of membranes and colour of amniotic fluid.
- Give Supportive care **D6-D7**.
- **Never leave the woman alone.**

MONITOR EVERY 4 HOURS:

- Cervical dilatation **D3** **D15**.
- Unless indicated, **do not** do vaginal examination more frequently than every 4 hours.
- Temperature.
- Pulse **B3**.
- Blood pressure **D23**.

ASSESS PROGRESS OF LABOUR

- After 8 hours if:
  → Contractions stronger and more frequent but
  → No progress in cervical dilatation with or without membranes ruptured.

- After 8 hours if:
  → no increase in contractions, and
  → membranes are not ruptured, and
  → no progress in cervical dilatation.

- Cervical dilatation 4 cm or greater.

TREAT AND ADVISE, IF REQUIRED

- Refer the woman urgently to hospital **B17**.

- Discharge the woman and advise her to return if:
  → pain/discomfort increases
  → vaginal bleeding
  → membranes rupture.

- Begin plotting the partograph **N5** and manage the woman as in active labour **D9**.

FIRST STAGE OF LABOUR: IN ACTIVE LABOUR

Use this chart when the woman is IN ACTIVE LABOUR, when cervix dilated 4 cm or more.

MONITOR EVERY 30 MINUTES:

- For emergency signs, using rapid assessment (RAM) **B3-B7**.
- Frequency, intensity and duration of contractions.
- Fetal heart rate **D14**.
- Mood and behaviour (distressed, anxious) **D6**.

- Record findings regularly in Labour record and Partograph **N4-N6**.
- Record time of rupture of membranes and colour of amniotic fluid.
- Give Supportive care **D6-D7**.
- **Never leave the woman alone.**

MONITOR EVERY 4 HOURS:

- Cervical dilatation **D3** **D15**.
- Unless indicated, **do not** do vaginal examination more frequently than every 4 hours.
- Temperature.
- Pulse **B3**.
- Blood pressure **D23**.

ASSESS PROGRESS OF LABOUR

- Partograph passes to the right of ALERT LINE.

- Partograph passes to the right of ACTION LINE.
- Cervix dilated 10 cm or bulging perineum.

TREAT AND ADVISE, IF REQUIRED

- Reassess woman and consider criteria for referral.
- Call senior person if available. Alert emergency transport services.
- Encourage woman to empty bladder.
- Ensure adequate hydration but omit solid foods.
- Encourage upright position and walking if woman wishes.
- Monitor intensively. Reassess in 2 hours and refer if no progress. If referral takes a long time, refer immediately (DO NOT wait to cross action line).

- **Refer urgently to hospital** **B17** unless birth is imminent.
- Manage as in *Second stage of labour* **D10-D11**.

Second stage of labour: deliver the baby and give immediate newborn care (1) — D10

SECOND STAGE OF LABOUR: DELIVER THE BABY AND GIVE IMMEDIATE NEWBORN CARE

Use this chart when cervix dilated 10 cm or bulging thin perineum and head visible.

MONITOR EVERY 5 MINUTES:

- For emergency signs, using rapid assessment (RAM) **B3-B7**.
- Frequency, intensity and duration of contractions.
- Fetal heart rate **D14**.
- Perineum thinning and bulging.
- Visible descent of fetal head or during contraction.
- Mood and behaviour (distressed, anxious) **D6**
- Record findings regularly in Labour record and Partograph **N4-N6**.
- Give Supportive care **D6-D7**.
- Never leave the woman alone.

DELIVER THE BABY

- Ensure all delivery equipment and supplies, including newborn resuscitation equipment, are available, and place of delivery is clean and warm (25°C) **L3**.

- Ensure bladder is empty.
- Assist the woman into a comfortable position of her choice, as upright as possible.
- Stay with her and offer her emotional and physical support **D10-D11**.

- Allow her to push as she wishes with contractions.

- Wait until head visible and perineum distending.
- Wash hands with clean water and soap. Put on sterile gloves just before delivery.
- See Universal precautions during labour and delivery **A4**.

TREAT AND ADVISE IF REQUIRED

- If unable to pass urine and bladder is full, empty bladder **B12**.
- **DO NOT** let her lie flat (horizontally) on her back.
- If the woman is distressed, encourage pain discomfort relief **D6**.

- **DO NOT** urge her to push.
- If, after 30 minutes of spontaneous expulsive efforts, the perineum does not begin to thin and stretch with contractions, do a vaginal examination to confirm full dilatation of cervix.
- If cervix is not fully dilated, await second stage. Place woman on her left side and discourage pushing. Encourage breathing technique **D6**.

- If second stage lasts for 2 hours or more without visible steady descent of the head, **refer urgently to hospital** **B17**.
- **DO NOT** routinely perform episiotomy.
- In the presence of physical obstruction due lesions or scar tissue in the perineum, a decision to perform episiotomy may be taken.
- If breech or other malpresentation, manage as on **D16**.

DELIVER THE BABY

- Ensure controlled delivery of the head:
  - → Keep one hand gently on the head as it advances with contractions.
  - → Support perineum with other hand and cover anus with pad held in position by side of hand during delivery.
  - → Leave the perineum visible (between thumb and first finger).
  - → Ask the mother to breathe steadily and not to push during delivery of the head.
  - → Encourage rapid breathing with mouth open.

- Feel gently around baby's neck for the cord.
- Check if the face is clear of mucus and membranes.

- Await spontaneous rotation of shoulders and delivery (within 1-2 minutes).
- Apply gentle downward pressure to deliver top shoulder.
- Then lift baby up, towards the mother's abdomen to deliver lower shoulder.
- Place baby on abdomen or in mother's arms.
- Note time of delivery.

- Thoroughly dry the baby immediately. Wipe eyes. Discard wet cloth.
- Assess baby's breathing while drying.
- If the baby is not crying, observe breathing:
  - → breathing well (chest rising)?
  - → not breathing or gasping?

- Palpate mother's abdomen to exclude a second baby.
- Give 10 IU oxytocin IM to the mother.
- Watch for vaginal bleeding.

- Change gloves.
- Clamp and cut the cord (1-3 minutes after birth):
  - → put ties tightly around the cord at 2 cm and 5 cm from baby's abdomen.
  - → cut between ties with sterile instrument.
  - → observe for oozing blood.

- Leave baby on the mother's chest in skin-to-skin contact. Place identification label.
- Cover the baby, cover the head with a hat.

- Encourage initiation of breastfeeding within the first hour after birth K2.

TREAT AND ADVISE IF REQUIRED

- If potentially damaging expulsive efforts, exert more pressure on perineum.
- Discard soiled pad to prevent infection.

- If cord present and loose, deliver the baby through the loop of cord or slip the cord over the baby's head; if cord is tight, clamp and cut cord, then unwind.
- Gently wipe face clean with gauze or cloth, if necessary.
- Routine suction or aspiration is not recommended. It should only be done in the presence of dense substances blocking the nose and mouth.

- If delay in delivery of shoulders:
  - → **DO NOT** panic but call for help and ask companion to assist
  - → Manage as in *Stuck shoulders* D17.
- If placing newborn on abdomen is not acceptable, or the mother cannot hold the baby, place the baby in a clean, warm, safe place close to the mother.

- **DO NOT** leave the baby wet - she/he will become cold.
- If the baby is not breathing or gasping (unless baby is dead, macerated, severely malformed):
  - → Stimulate by rubbing the back 2 to 3 times.
  - → Cut cord quickly: transfer to a firm, warm surface; start Newborn resuscitation K11.
- Routine suction or aspiration is not recommended. It should only be done in the presence of dense substances blocking the nose and mouth.
- CALL FOR HELP - one person should care for the mother.

- If second baby, **DO NOT** give oxytocin now. **GET HELP**.
- Deliver the second baby. Manage as in *Multiple pregnancy* D18.
- If heavy bleeding, repeat oxytocin 10-IU-IM B5.

- If blood oozing, place a second tie between the skin and the first tie.
- **DO NOT** apply any substance to the stump.
- **DO NOT** bandage or bind the stump.

- If room cool (less than 25°C), use additional blanket to cover the mother and baby.

- If HIV-infected mother has chosen replacement feeding, feed accordingly.
- Check ARV treatment needed G6, G9.

Second stage of labour: deliver the baby and give immediate newborn care (2) D11

Third stage of labour: deliver the placenta D12

THIRD STAGE OF LABOUR: DELIVER THE PLACENTA

Use this chart for care of the woman between birth of the baby and delivery of placenta.

MONITOR MOTHER EVERY 5 MINUTES:

- For emergency signs, using rapid assessment (RAM) **B3-B7**.
- Feel if uterus is well contracted.
- Mood and behaviour (distressed, anxious) **D6**.
- Time since third stage began (time since birth).

- Record findings, treatments and procedures in *Labour record and Partograph* **N4-N6**.
- Give *Supportive care* **D6-D7**.
- **Never leave the woman alone.**

MONITOR BABY EVERY 15 MINUTES:

- Breathing: listen for grunting, look for chest in-drawing and fast breathing **J2**.
- Warmth: check to see if feet are cold to touch **J2**.

DELIVER THE PLACENTA

- Ensure 10-IU oxytocin IM is given **D11**.
- Await strong uterine contraction (2-3 minutes) and deliver placenta by **controlled cord traction**:
  → Place side of one hand (usually left) above symphysis pubis with palm facing towards the mother's umbilicus. This applies counter traction to the uterus during controlled cord traction. At the same time, apply steady, sustained controlled cord traction.
  → If placenta does not descend during 30-40 seconds of controlled cord traction, release both cord traction and counter traction on the abdomen and wait until the uterus is well contracted again. Then repeat controlled cord traction with counter traction.
  → As the placenta is coming out, catch in both hands to prevent tearing of the membranes.
  → If the membranes do not slip out spontaneously, gently twist them into a rope and move them up and down to assist separation without tearing them.

- Check that placenta and membranes are complete.

TREAT AND ADVISE IF REQUIRED

- If, after 30 minutes of giving oxytocin, the placenta is not delivered and the woman is NOT bleeding:
  → Empty bladder **B12**
  → Encourage breastfeeding
  → Repeat controlled cord traction.
- If woman is bleeding, manage as on **B5**
- If placenta is not delivered in another 30 minutes (1 hour after delivery):
  → Remove placenta manually **B11**
  → Give appropriate IM/IV antibiotic **B15**.
- If in 1 hour unable to remove placenta:
  → Refer the woman to hospital **B17**
  → Insert an IV line and give fluids with 20 IU of oxytocin at 30 drops per minute during transfer **B9**.
- **DO NOT** exert excessive traction on the cord.
- **DO NOT** squeeze or push the uterus to deliver the placenta.

- If placenta is incomplete:
  → Remove placental fragments manually **B11**.
  → Give appropriate IM/IV antibiotic **B15**.

DELIVER THE PLACENTA

- Check that uterus is well contracted and there is no heavy bleeding.
- Repeat check every 5 minutes.

TREAT AND ADVISE IF REQUIRED

- If heavy bleeding **B5**:
  → Massage uterus to expel clots if any, until it is hard **B10**.
  → Give oxytocin 10 IU IM **B10**.
  → Call for help.
  → Start an IV line **B9**, add 20 IU of oxytocin to IV fluids and give at 60 drops per minute **B10**.
  → Empty the bladder **B12**.
- If bleeding persists and uterus is soft:
  → Continue massaging uterus until it is hard.
  → Apply bimanual or aortic compression **B10**.
  → Continue IV fluids with 20 IU of oxytocin at 30 drops per minute.
  → **Refer woman urgently to hospital B17**.

- Examine perineum, lower vagina and vulva for tears.

- If third degree tear (involving rectum or anus), **refer urgently to hospital B17**.
- For other tears: apply pressure over the tear with a sterile pad or gauze and put legs together.
- Check after 5 minutes. If bleeding persists, repair the tear **B12**.

- Collect, estimate and record blood loss throughout third stage and immediately afterwards.

- If blood loss ≈ 250 ml, but bleeding has stopped:
  → Plan to keep the woman in the facility for 24 hours.
  → Monitor intensively (every 30 minutes) for 4 hours:
    → Blood pressure, pulse
    → vaginal bleeding
    → uterus, to make sure it is well contracted.
  → Assist the woman when she first walks after resting and recovering.
  → If not possible to observe at the facility, **refer to hospital B17**.

- Clean the woman and the area beneath her. Put sanitary pad or folded clean cloth under her buttocks to collect blood. Help her to change clothes if necessary.

- Keep the mother and baby in delivery room for a minimum of one hour after delivery of placenta.

- Dispose of placenta in the correct, safe and culturally appropriate manner.

- If disposing placenta:
  → Use gloves when handling placenta.
  → Put placenta into a bag and place it into a leak-proof container.
  → Always carry placenta in a leak-proof container.
  → Incinerate the placenta or bury it at least 10 m away from a water source, in a 2 m deep pit.

Third stage of labour: deliver the placenta

Respond to problems during labour and delivery (1) ▶ If FHR <120 or >160bpm **D14**

CHILDBIRTH: LABOUR, DELIVERY AND IMMEDIATE POSTPARTUM CARE

RESPOND TO PROBLEMS DURING LABOUR AND DELIVERY

ASK, CHECK RECORD	LOOK, LISTEN, FEEL	SIGNS	CLASSIFY	TREAT AND ADVISE

IF FETAL HEART RATE (FHR) <120 OR >160 BEATS PER MINUTE

	LOOK, LISTEN, FEEL	SIGNS	CLASSIFY	TREAT AND ADVISE
	■ Position the woman on her left side. ■ If membranes have ruptured, look at vulva for prolapsed cord. ■ See if liquor was meconium stained. ■ Repeat FHR count after 15 minutes	■ Cord seen at vulva.	**PROLAPSED CORD**	■ Manage urgently as on **D15**.
		■ FHR remains >160 or <120 after 30 minutes observation.	**BABY NOT WELL**	■ If early labour: → **Refer the woman urgently to hospital B17** → Keep her lying on her left side. ■ If late labour: → Call for help during delivery → Monitor after every contraction. If FHR does not return to normal in 15 minutes explain to the woman (and her companion) that the baby may not be well **D15**. → Prepare for newborn resuscitation **K11**.
		■ FHR returns to normal.	**BABY WELL**	■ Monitor FHR every 15 minutes.

▼ **Next:** If prolapsed cord

IF PROLAPSED CORD

The cord is visible outside the vagina or can be felt in the vagina below the presenting part.

ASK, CHECK RECORD	LOOK, LISTEN, FEEL	SIGNS	CLASSIFY	TREAT
	■ Look at or feel the cord gently for pulsations. ■ Check for FHR ■ Feel for transverse lie. ■ Do vaginal examination to determine status of labour.	■ Transverse lie	OBSTRUCTED LABOUR	■ Refer urgently to hospital B17.
		■ Cord is pulsating	FETUS ALIVE	**If early labour:** ■ Push the head or presenting part out of the pelvis and hold it above the brim/pelvis with your hand on the abdomen until caesarean section is performed. ■ Instruct assistant (family, staff) to position the woman's buttocks higher than the shoulder. ■ Refer urgently to hospital B17. ■ If transfer not possible, allow labour to continue. **If late labour:** ■ Call for additional help if possible (for mother and baby). ■ Prepare for Newborn resuscitation K11. ■ Expedite delivery. If not possible, refer urgently to hospital.
		■ Cord is not pulsating	FETUS PROBABLY DEAD	■ Explain to the woman and companion that baby may not be well.

 Next: If breech presentation

Respond to problems during labour and delivery (2) ▶ If prolapsed cord

D15

Respond to problems during labour and delivery (3) ▶ If breech presentation

D16

IF BREECH PRESENTATION

LOOK, LISTEN, FEEL

- On external examination fetal head felt in fundus.
- Soft body part (leg or buttocks) felt on vaginal examination.
- Legs or buttocks presenting at perineum.

SIGNS	TREAT
■ If early labour	■ **Refer urgently to hospital** B17.
■ If late labour	■ Call for additional help. ■ Confirm full dilatation of the cervix by vaginal examination D3. ■ Ensure bladder is empty. If unable to empty bladder see Empty bladder B12. ■ Prepare for newborn resuscitation K11. ■ Deliver the baby: → Assist the woman into a position that will allow the baby to hang down during delivery, for example, propped up with buttocks at edge of bed or onto her hands and knees (all fours position). → **DO NOT** routinely perform episiotomy. → Allow buttocks, trunk and shoulders to deliver spontaneously during contractions. → After delivery of the shoulders allow the baby to hang until next contraction.
■ If the head does not deliver after several contractions	■ Place the baby astride your left forearm with limbs hanging on each side. ■ Place the middle and index fingers of the left hand over the malar cheek bones on either side to apply gentle downwards pressure to aid flexion of head. ■ Keeping the left hand as described, place the index and ring fingers of the right hand over the baby's shoulders and the middle finger on the baby's head to gently aid flexion until the hairline is visible. ■ When the hairline is visible, raise the baby in upward and forward direction towards the mother's abdomen until the nose and mouth are free. The assistant gives supra pubic pressure during the period to maintain flexion.
■ If trapped arms or shoulders	■ Feel the baby's chest for arms. If not felt: ■ Hold the baby gently with hands around each thigh and thumbs on sacrum. ■ Gently guiding the baby down, turn the baby, keeping the back uppermost until the shoulder which was posterior (below) is now anterior (at the top) and the arm is released. ■ Then turn the baby back, again keeping the back uppermost to deliver the other arm. ■ Then proceed with delivery of head as described above.
■ If trapped head (and baby is dead)	■ Proceed with delivery of head as described above. ■ **NEVER** pull on the breech ■ **DO NOT** allow the woman to push until the cervix is fully dilated. Pushing too soon may cause the head to be trapped.

Next: If stuck shoulders

IF STUCK SHOULDERS (SHOULDER DYSTOCIA)

SIGNS	TREAT
■ Fetal head is delivered, but shoulders are stuck and cannot be delivered.	■ Call for additional help. ■ Prepare for newborn resuscitation K11. ■ Explain the problem to the woman and her companion. ■ Ask the woman to lie on her back while gripping her legs tightly flexed against her chest, with knees wide apart. Ask the companion or other helper to keep the legs in that position. ■ **DO NOT** routinely perform episiotomy. ■ Ask an assistant to apply continuous pressure downwards, with the palm of the hand on the abdomen directly above the pubic area, while you maintain continuous downward traction on the fetal head.
■ If the shoulders are still not delivered and surgical help is not available immediately.	■ Remain calm and explain to the woman that you need her cooperation to try another position. ■ Assist her to adopt a kneeling on "all fours" position and ask her companion to hold her steady - this simple change of position is sometimes sufficient to dislodge the impacted shoulder and achieve delivery. ■ Introduce the right hand into the vagina along the posterior curve of the sacrum. ■ Attempt to deliver the posterior shoulder or arm using pressure from the finger of the right hand to hook the posterior shoulder and arm downwards and forwards through the vagina. ■ Complete the rest of delivery as normal. ■ If not successful, **refer urgently to hospital** B17. **DO NOT** pull excessively on the head.

 Next: If multiple births

Respond to problems during labour and delivery (5) ▶ If multiple births

D18

CHILDBIRTH: LABOUR, DELIVERY AND IMMEDIATE POSTPARTUM CARE

IF MULTIPLE BIRTHS

SIGNS	TREAT
■ Prepare for delivery	■ Prepare delivery room and equipment for birth of 2 or more babies. Include: → more warm cloths → two sets of cord ties and razor blades → resuscitation equipment for 2 babies. ■ Arrange for a helper to assist you with the births and care of the babies.
■ Second stage of labour	■ Deliver the first baby following the usual procedure. Resuscitate if necessary. Label her/him Twin 1. ■ Ask helper to attend to the first baby. ■ Palpate uterus immediately to determine the lie of the second baby. If transverse or oblique lie, gently turn the baby by abdominal manipulation to head or breech presentation. ■ Check the presentation by vaginal examination. Check the fetal heart rate. ■ Await the return of strong contractions and spontaneous rupture of the second bag of membranes, usually within 1 hour of birth of first baby, but may be longer. ■ Stay with the woman and continue monitoring her and the fetal heart rate intensively. ■ Remove wet cloths from underneath her. If feeling chilled, cover her. ■ When the membranes rupture, perform vaginal examination **D3** to check for prolapsed cord. If present, see Prolapsed cord **D15**. ■ When strong contractions restart, ask the mother to bear down when she feels ready. ■ Deliver the second baby. Resuscitate if necessary. Label her/him Twin 2. ■ After cutting the cord, ask the helper to attend to the second baby. ■ Palpate the uterus for a third baby. If a third baby is felt, proceed as described above. If no third baby is felt, go to third stage of labour. ■ **DO NOT** attempt to deliver the placenta until all the babies are born. ■ **DO NOT** give the mother oxytocin until after the birth of all babies.
■ Third stage of labour	■ Give oxytocin 10 IU IM after making sure there is not another baby. ■ When the uterus is well contracted, deliver the placenta and membranes by applying traction to all cords together **D12-D23**. ■ Before and after delivery of the placenta and membranes, observe closely for vaginal bleeding because this woman is at greater risk of postpartum haemorrhage. ■ If placenta incomplete, see **B11**. ■ Examine the placenta and membranes for completeness. There may be one large placenta with 2 umbilical cords, or a separate placenta with an umbilical cord for each baby.
■ Immediate postpartum care	■ Monitor intensively as risk of bleeding is increased. ■ Provide immediate Postpartum care **D19-D20**. ■ In addition: → Keep mother in health centre at least 24 hours after birth. → Plan to measure haemoglobin postpartum if possible → Give special support for care and feeding of babies **J11** and **K4**.

▼ **Next:** Care of the mother and newborn within first hour of delivery of placenta

CARE OF THE MOTHER AND NEWBORN WITHIN FIRST HOUR OF DELIVERY OF PLACENTA

Use this chart for woman and newborn during the first hour after complete delivery of placenta.

MONITOR MOTHER EVERY 15 MINUTES:

- For emergency signs, using rapid assessment (RAM) **B3-B7**.
- Feel if uterus is hard and round.

- Record findings, treatments and procedures in *Labour record and Partograph* **N4-N6**.
- Keep mother and baby in delivery room - **do not separate them**.
- **Never leave the woman and newborn alone.**

MONITOR BABY EVERY 15 MINUTES:

- Breathing: listen for grunting, look for chest in-drawing and fast breathing **J2**.
- Warmth: check to see if feet are cold to touch **J2**.
- Check colour, umbilical cord for oozing, sucking/feeding.

CARE OF MOTHER AND NEWBORN

WOMAN
- Assess the amount of vaginal bleeding.
- Encourage the woman to eat and drink.
- Ask the companion to stay with the mother.
- Encourage the woman to pass urine.

NEWBORN
- Wipe the eyes.
- Apply antiseptic eye drops or ointment (e.g. tetracycline ointment) to both eyes once, according to national guidelines.
- DO NOT wash away the eye antimicrobial.
- If blood or meconium, wipe off with wet cloth and dry.
- DO NOT remove vernix or bathe the baby.
- Continue keeping the baby warm and in skin-to-skin contact with the mother.
- Encourage the mother to initiate breastfeeding when baby shows signs of readiness. Offer her help.
- DO NOT give artificial teats or pre-lacteal feeds to the newborn: no water, sugar water, or local feeds.

- Examine the mother and newborn one hour after delivery of placenta.
- Use *Assess the mother after delivery* **D21** and *Examine the newborn* **J2-J8**.

INTERVENTIONS, IF REQUIRED

- If pad soaked in less than 5 minutes, or constant trickle of blood, manage as on **D22**.
- If uterus soft, manage as on **B10**.
- If bleeding from a perineal tear, repair if required **B12** or **refer to hospital B17**.

- If breathing with difficulty — grunting, chest in-drawing or fast breathing, examine the baby as on **J2-J8**.
- If feet are cold to touch or mother and baby are separated:
- Ensure the room is warm. Cover mother and baby with a blanket
  → Reassess in 1 hour. If still cold, measure temperature. If less than 36.5°C, manage as on **K9**.
- If unable to initiate breastfeeding (mother has complications):
  → Plan for alternative feeding method **K5-K6**.
  → If mother HIV-infected: assess risk of HIV infection infant and prescribe appropriate prophylaxis (either single drug NVP or dual prophylaxis with NVP and AZT) **G9**.
  → Support the mother's choice of newborn feeding **G8**.
- If baby is stillborn or dead, give supportive care to mother and her family **D24**.

- **Refer to hospital** now if woman had serious complications at admission or during delivery but was in late labour.

Care of the mother and newborn within first hour of delivery of placenta   **D19**

Care of the mother one hour after delivery of placenta D20

CARE OF THE MOTHER ONE HOUR AFTER DELIVERY OF PLACENTA

Use this chart for continuous care of the mother until discharge. See **J10** for care of the baby.

MONITOR MOTHER AT 2, 3 AND 4 HOURS, THEN EVERY 4 HOURS:

- For emergency signs, using rapid assessment (RAM) **B4-B7**.
- Feel uterus if hard and round.

- Record findings, treatments and procedures in *Labour record and Partograph* **N4-N6**.
- Keep the mother and baby together.
- **Never leave the woman and newborn alone.**
- **DO NOT** discharge before 24 hours.

CARE OF MOTHER

- Accompany the mother and baby to ward.
- Advise on *Postpartum care and hygiene* **D26**.
- Ensure the mother has sanitary napkins or clean material to collect vaginal blood.
- Encourage the mother to eat, drink and rest.
- Ensure the room is warm (25°C).

- Ask the mother's companion to watch her and call for help if bleeding or pain increases, if mother feels dizzy or has severe headaches, visual disturbance or epigastric distress.

- Encourage the mother to empty her bladder and ensure that she has passed urine.

- Check record and give any treatment or prophylaxis which is due.
- Advise the mother on postpartum care and nutrition **D26**.
- Advise when to seek care **D28**.
- Counsel on return to fertility, healthy timing and spacing of pregnancy and family planning options **D27**.
- Repeat examination of the mother before discharge using *Assess the mother after delivery* **D21**. For baby, see **J2-J8**.

INTERVENTIONS, IF REQUIRED

- Make sure the woman has someone with her and they know when to call for help.
- If HIV-infected: give her appropriate treatment **G6**, **G9**.

- If heavy vaginal bleeding, palpate the uterus.
  → If uterus not firm, massage the fundus to make it contract and expel any clots **B6**.
  → If pad is soaked in less than 5 minutes, manage as on **B5**.
  → If bleeding is from perineal tear, repair or refer to hospital **B17**.

- If the mother cannot pass urine or the bladder is full (swelling over lower abdomen) and she is uncomfortable, help her by gently pouring water on vulva.
- **DO NOT** catheterize unless you have to.

- If tubal ligation or IUD desired, make plans before discharge.

ASSESS THE MOTHER AFTER DELIVERY

After an uncomplicated vaginal birth in a health facility, healthy mothers and newborns should receive care in the facility for at least 24 hours after birth.
Use this chart to examine the mother the first time after delivery (at 1 hour after delivery or later) and for discharge.
For examining the newborn use the chart on J2-J8.

ASK, CHECK RECORD

- Check record:
  → bleeding more than 250 ml?
  → completeness of placenta and membranes?
  → complications during delivery or postpartum?
  → special treatment needs?
  → needs tubal ligation or IUD?
- How are you feeling?
- Do you have any pains?
- Do you have any concerns?
- How is your baby?
- How do your breasts feel?

LOOK, LISTEN, FEEL

- Measure temperature.
- Measure blood pressure and pulse
- Feel the uterus. Is it hard and round?
- Look for vaginal bleeding
- Look at perineum.
  → Is there a tear or cut?
  → Is it red, swollen or draining pus?
- Look for conjunctival pallor.
- Look for palmar pallor.

SIGNS

- Uterus hard.
- Little bleeding.
- No perineal problem.
- No pallor.
- No fever.
- Blood pressure normal.
- Pulse normal.

CLASSIFY

MOTHER WELL

TREAT AND ADVISE

- Keep the mother at the facility for 24 hours after delivery.
- Ensure preventive measures D25.
- Advise on postpartum care and hygiene D26.
- Counsel on nutrition D26.
- Counsel on birth spacing and family planning D27.
- Advise on when to seek care and next routine postpartum visit D28.
- Reassess for discharge.
- Continue any treatments initiated earlier.
- If tubal ligation desired, refer to hospital within 7 days of delivery. If IUD desired, refer to appropriate services within 48 hours.

▼ **Next:** Respond to problems immediately postpartum
If no problems, go to page D25.

Assess the mother after delivery D21

Respond to problems during and immediately after childbirth (1)

D22

CHILDBIRTH: LABOUR, DELIVERY AND IMMEDIATE POSTPARTUM CARE

ASK, CHECK RECORD	LOOK, LISTEN, FEEL	SIGNS	CLASSIFY	TREAT AND ADVISE
IF VAGINAL BLEEDING				
	■ A pad is soaked in less than ■ 5 minutes.	■ More than 1 pad soaked in 5 minutes ■ Uterus not hard and not round	HEAVY BLEEDING	■ See **B5** for treatment. ■ Refer urgently to hospital **B17**.
IF FEVER (TEMPERATURE >38°C)				
■ Time since rupture of membranes ■ Abdominal pain ■ Chills	■ Repeat temperature measurement after 2 hours ■ If temperature is still >38°C → Look for abnormal vaginal discharge. → Listen to fetal heart rate → feel lower abdomen for tenderness	■ Temperature still >38°C and any of: → Chills → Foul-smelling vaginal discharge → Low abdomen tenderness → FHR remains > 160 after 30 minutes of observation. → rupture of membranes >18 hours	UTERINE AND FETAL INFECTION	■ Insert an IV line and give fluids rapidly **B6** ■ Give appropriate IM/IV antibiotics **B15**. ■ If baby and placenta delivered: → Give oxytocin 10 IU IM **B10**. ■ Refer woman urgently to hospital **B17** ■ Assess the newborn **J2-J8**. Treat if any sign of infection.
		■ Temperature still >38°C	RISK OF UTERINE AND FETAL INFECTION	■ Encourage woman to drink plenty of fluids. ■ Measure temperature every 4 hours. ■ If temperature persists for >12 hours, is very high or rises rapidly, give appropriate antibiotic and refer to hospital **B15**.
IF PERINEAL TEAR OR EPISIOTOMY				
	■ Is there bleeding from the tear or episiotomy ■ Does it extend to anus or rectum?	■ Tear extending to anus or rectum.	THIRD DEGREE TEAR	■ Refer woman urgently to hospital **B15**.
		■ Perineal tear ■ Episiotomy	SMALL PERINEAL TEAR	■ If bleeding persists, repair the tear or episiotomy **B12**.

Next: If elevated diastolic blood pressure

IF ELEVATED DIASTOLIC BLOOD PRESSURE

ASK, CHECK RECORD	LOOK, LISTEN, FEEL	SIGNS	CLASSIFY	TREAT AND ADVISE
	■ If diastolic blood pressure is ≥90 mmHg, repeat after 1 hour rest. ■ If diastolic blood pressure is still ≥90 mmHg, ask the woman if she has: → severe headache → blurred vision → epigastric pain and → check protein in urine.	■ Diastolic blood pressure ≥110 mmHg and 3+ proteinuria, or ■ Diastolic blood pressure ≥90 mmHg on two readings and 2+ proteinuria, and any of: → severe headache → blurred vision → epigastric pain.	**SEVERE PRE-ECLAMPSIA**	■ Give magnesium sulphate B13. ■ If in early labour or postpartum, **refer urgently to hospital** B17. ■ **If late labour:** → continue magnesium sulphate treatment B13 → monitor blood pressure every hour. → **DO NOT** give ergometrine after delivery. ■ **Refer urgently to hospital after delivery** B17.
		■ Diastolic blood pressure 90-110 mmHg on two readings. ■ 2+ proteinuria (on admission).	**PRE-ECLAMPSIA**	■ If early labour, **refer urgently to hospital** B17. ■ If late labour: → monitor blood pressure every hour B9 → **DO NOT** give ergometrine after delivery. ■ If blood pressure remains elevated after delivery, **refer to hospital** E17.
		■ Diastolic blood pressure ≥90 mmHg on 2 readings.	**HYPERTENSION**	■ Monitor blood pressure every hour. ■ **Do not** give ergometrine after delivery. ■ If blood pressure remains elevated after delivery, **refer woman to hospital** E17.

 Next: If pallor on screening, check for anaemia

Respond to problems during and immediately after childbirth. (2)

Respond to problems immediately postpartum

D24

CHILDBIRTH: LABOUR, DELIVERY AND IMMEDIATE POSTPARTUM CARE

ASK, CHECK RECORD	LOOK, LISTEN, FEEL	SIGNS	CLASSIFY	TREAT AND ADVISE
IF PALLOR ON SCREENING, CHECK FOR ANAEMIA				
■ Bleeding during labour, delivery or postpartum.	■ Measure haemoglobin, if possible. ■ Look for conjunctival pallor. ■ Look for palmar pallor. If pallor: → Is it severe pallor? → Some pallor? → Count number of breaths in → 1 minute	■ Haemoglobin <7 g/dl. **AND/OR** ■ Severe palmar and conjunctival pallor or ■ Any pallor with >30 breaths per minute.	**SEVERE ANAEMIA**	■ If early labour or postpartum, **refer urgently to hospital** **B17**. ■ **If late labour:** → monitor intensively **D9**. → minimize blood loss → **refer urgently to hospital after delivery** **B17**.
		■ Any bleeding. ■ Haemoglobin 7-11 g/dl. ■ Palmar or conjunctival pallor.	**MODERATE ANAEMIA**	■ Check haemoglobin after 3 days. ■ Give double dose of iron for 3 months **F3**. ■ Follow up in 4 weeks.
		■ Haemoglobin >11 g/dl ■ No pallor.	**NO ANAEMIA**	■ Give iron/folate for 3 months **F3**.
IF MOTHER SEVERELY ILL OR SEPARATED FROM THE BABY				
				■ Teach mother to express breast milk every 3 hours **K5**. ■ Help her to express breast milk if necessary. Ensure baby receives mother's milk **K8**. ■ Help her to establish or re-establish breastfeeding as soon as possible. See **K2-K3**.
IF BABY STILLBORN OR DEAD				
				■ Give supportive care: → Inform the parents as soon as possible after the baby's death. → Show the baby to the mother, give the baby to the mother to hold, where culturally appropriate. → Offer the parents and family to be with the dead baby in privacy as long as they need. → Discuss with them the events before the death and the possible causes of death. ■ Advise the mother on breast care **K8**. ■ Counsel on appropriate family planning method **D27**. ■ Record the event. Complete the perinatal death certificate **N7**.

▼ Next: Give preventive measures

GIVE PREVENTIVE MEASURES

Ensure that all are given before discharge.

ASSESS, CHECK RECORDS

- Check RPR status in records.
- If no RPR during this pregnancy, do the RPR test `L5`.

- Check tetanus toxoid (TT) immunization status.
- Check when last dose of mebendazole was given.

- Check woman's supply of prescribed dose of iron/folate.

- Ask whether woman and baby are sleeping under insecticide treated bednet.
- Counsel and advise all women.

- Record all treatments given `N6`.
- Record findings on home-based record.

- Check HIV status in records.

TREAT AND ADVISE

- If RPR positive:
  → Treat woman and the partner with benzathine penicillin `F6`.
  → Treat the newborn `K12`.

- Give tetanus toxoid if due `F2`.
- Give mebendazole once in 6 months `F3`.

- Give 3 month's supply of iron and counsel on adherence `F2`.
- Vitamin A in postpartum women is not recommended for the prevention of maternal and infant morbidity and mortality.

- Encourage sleeping under insecticide treated bednet `F4`.
- Advise on postpartum care `D26`.
- Counsel on nutrition `D26`.
- Counsel on birth spacing and family planning `D27`.
- Counsel on breastfeeding `K2`.
- Counsel on safer sex including use of condoms `G2`.
- Advise on routine and follow-up postpartum visits `D28`.
- Advise on danger signs `D28`.
- Discuss how to prepare for an emergency in postpartum `D28`.
- Counsel of continued abstinence from tobacco, alcohol and drugs `D26`.

- If HIV-infected:
  → Support adherence to ARV `G6`.
  → Treat the newborn `G9`.
- If HIV test not done, the result of the latest test not known or if tested HIV-negative in early pregnancy, offer her the rapid HIV test `C6`, `E5`, `L6`.

Give preventive measures

D25

Advise on postpartum care   D26

ADVISE ON POSTPARTUM CARE

Advise on postpartum care and hygiene

- Advise and explain to the woman:
- To always have someone near her for the first 24 hours to respond to any change in her condition.
- Not to insert anything into the vagina.
- To have enough rest and sleep.
- The importance of washing to prevent infection of the mother and her baby:
  - → wash hands before handling baby
  - → wash perineum daily and after faecal excretion
  - → change perineal pads every 4 to 6 hours, or more frequently if heavy lochia
  - → wash used pads or dispose of them safely
  - → wash the body daily.
- To avoid sexual intercourse until the perineal wound heals.
- To sleep with the baby under an insecticide-treated bednet.

Counsel on nutrition

- Advise the woman to eat a greater amount and variety of healthy foods, such as meat, fish, oils, nuts, seeds, cereals, beans, vegetables, cheese, milk, to help her feel well and strong (give examples of types of food and how much to eat).
- Reassure the mother that she can eat any normal foods – these will not harm the breastfeeding baby.
- Spend more time on nutrition counselling with very thin women and adolescents.
- Determine if there are important taboos about foods which are nutritionally healthy. Advise the woman against these taboos.
- Talk to family members such as partner and mother-in-law, to encourage them to help ensure the woman eats enough and avoids hard physical work.

Counsel on Substance Abuse

- Advise the woman to continue abstinence from tobacco
- Do not take any drugs or medications for tobacco cessation
- Talk to family members such as partner and mother-in-law, to encourage them to help ensure the woman avoids second-hand smoke exposure, alcohol and drugs.

COUNSEL ON BIRTH SPACING AND FAMILY PLANNING

Counsel on the importance of family planning

- If appropriate, ask the woman if she would like her partner or another family member to be included in the counselling session.
- Explain that after birth, if she has sex and is not exclusively breastfeeding, she can become pregnant as soon as 4 weeks after delivery. Therefore it is important to start thinking early about what family planning method they will use.
  → Ask about plans for having more children. If she (and her partner) want more children, advise that waiting at least 2 years before trying to become pregnant again is good for the mother and for the baby's health.
  → Information on when to start a method after delivery will vary depending on whether a woman is breastfeeding or not.
  → Make arrangements for the woman to see a family planning counsellor, or counsel her directly (see the *Decision-making tool for family planning providers and clients* for information on methods and on the counselling process).
- Councel on safer sex including use of condoms for dual protection from sexually transmitted infection (STI) or HIV and pregnancy. Promote their use, especially if at risk for sexually transmitted infection (STI) or HIV G2.
- For HIV-infected women, see G4 for family planning considerations
- Her partner can decide to have a vasectomy (male sterilization) at any time.

Method options for the non-breastfeeding woman

Can be used immediately postpartum	Condoms Progestogen-only oral contraceptives Progestogen-only injectables Implant Spermicide Female sterilization (within 7 days or delay 6 weeks) Copper IUD or levonorgestrel-releasing intrauterine device (LNG-IUD) (immediately following expulsion of placenta or within 48 hours)
Delay 3 weeks	Combined oral contraceptives Combined injectables Fertility awareness methods

Lactational amenorrhoea method (LAM)

- A breastfeeding woman is protected from pregnancy only if:
  → she is no more than 6 months postpartum, and
  → she is breastfeeding exclusively (8 or more times a day, including at least once at night: no daytime feedings more than 4 hours apart and no night feedings more than 6 hours apart; no complementary foods or fluids), and
  → her menstrual cycle has not returned.

- A breastfeeding woman can also choose any other family planning method, either to use alone or together with LAM.

Method options for the breastfeeding woman

Can be used immediately postpartum	Lactational amenorrhoea method (LAM) Condoms Spermicide Female sterilisation (within 7 days or delay 6 weeks) Copper IUD or levonorgestrel-releasing intrauterine device (LNG-IUD) (within 48 hours or delay 4 weeks)
6 weeks postpartum	Breastfeeding women who are < 6 weeks postpartum can generally use progestogen-only pills (POPs) and levonorgestrel (LNG) and etonogestrel (ETG) implants. Breastfeeding women who are < 6 weeks postpartum generally should not use progestogen-only injectables (POIs) (Depot medroxyprogesterone acetate – DMPA or Norethisterone enanthate - NET-EN).
6 weeks to < 6 months	Breastfeeding women who are >= 6 weeks to < 6 months postpartum can generally use progestogen-only pills (POPs), POIs and levonorgestrel (LNG) and etonogestrel (ETG) implants.
6 months	Breastfeeding women who are >= 6 weeks to < 6 months postpartum can generally use progestogen-only pills (POPs), POIs and levonorgestrel (LNG) and etonogestrel (ETG) implants.

Advise on when to return

D28

ADVISE ON WHEN TO RETURN

Use this chart for advising on postnatal care after delivery in health facility on D21 or E2. For newborn babies see the schedule on K14.
Encourage woman to bring her partner or family member to at least one visit.

Routine postnatal contacts

FIRST CONTACT: within 24 hours after childbirth.
SECOND CONTACT: on day 3 (48-72 hours)
THIRD CONTACT: between day 7 and 14 after birth.
FINAL POSTNATAL CONTACT (CLINIC VISIT): at 6 weeks after birth

Follow-up visits for problems

If the problem was:	Return in:
Fever	2 days
Lower urinary tract infection	2 days
Perineal infection or pain	2 days
Hypertension	1 week
Urinary incontinence	1 week
Severe anaemia	2 weeks
Postpartum blues	2 weeks
HIV-infected	2 weeks
Moderate anaemia	4 weeks
If treated in hospital for any complication	According to hospital instructions or according to national guidelines, but no later than in 2 weeks.

Advise on danger signs

Advise to go to a hospital or health centre immediately, day or night, WITHOUT WAITING, if any of the following signs:
- vaginal bleeding:
  → more than 2 or 3 pads soaked in 20-30 minutes after delivery **OR**
  → bleeding increases rather than decreases after delivery.
- convulsions.
- Headache with blurred vision.
- fast or difficult breathing.
- fever and too weak to get out of bed.
- severe abdominal pain.
- calf pain, redness or swelling, shortness of breath or chest pain.

Go to health centre **as soon as possible** if any of the following signs:
- fever
- abdominal pain
- feels ill
- breasts swollen, red or tender breasts, or sore nipple
- urine dribbling or pain on micturition
- pain in the perineum or draining pus
- foul-smelling lochia
- severe depression or suicidal behaviour (ideas or attempts)

Discuss how to prepare for an emergency in postpartum

- Advise to always have someone near for at least 24 hours after delivery to respond to any change in condition.
- Discuss with woman and her partner and family about emergency issues:
  → where to go if danger signs
  → how to reach the hospital
  → costs involved
  → family and community support.
- Discuss home visits: in addition to the scheduled routine postnatal contacts, which can occur in clinics or at home, the mother and newborn may receive postnatal home visits by community health workers.
- Advise the woman to ask for help from the community, if needed I1-I3.
- Advise the woman to bring her home-based maternal record to the health centre, even for an

HOME DELIVERY BY SKILLED ATTENDANT

Use these instructions if you are attending delivery at home.

Preparation for home delivery

- Check emergency arrangements.
- Keep emergency transport arrangements up-to-date.
- Carry with you all essential drugs `B17`, records, and the delivery kit.
- Ensure that the family prepares, as on `C18`.

Delivery care

- Follow the labour and delivery procedures `D2-D28` `K11`.
- Observe universal precautions `A4`.
- Give **Supportive care**. Involve the companion in care and support `D6-D7`.
- Maintain the partograph and labour record `N4-N6`.
- Provide newborn care `J2-J8`.
- In settings with high neonatal mortality apply 7.1% chlorhexidine digluconate (gel or liquid) to the umbilical stump daily for the first week of life.
- **Refer to facility as soon as possible if any abnormal finding in mother or baby** `B17` `K14`.

Immediate postpartum care of mother

- Stay with the woman for first two hours after delivery of placenta `D13`.
- Examine the mother before leaving her `D21`.
- Advise on postpartum care, nutrition and family planning `D26-D27`.
- Ensure that someone will stay with the mother for the first 24 hours.

Postnatal care of newborn

- Stay until baby has had the first breastfeed and help the mother good positioning and attachment `K3`.
- Advise on breastfeeding `K2-K4`.
- Examine the baby before leaving `J2-J8`.
- Immunize the baby if possible `K13`.
- Advise on newborn care `K9-K10` `M6-M7`.
- Advise the family about danger signs and when and where to seek care `K14`.
- If possible, return within a day to check the mother and baby.
- Advise on the first postnatal contact for the mother and the baby which should be as early as possible within 24 hours of birth `K14`.

For both

- Return after 24 hours and on day 3 after delivery.
- Complete home-based record.

POSTPARTUM CARE

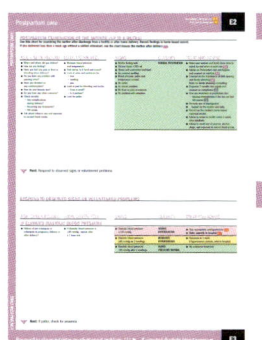

E2 **POSTPARTUM EXAMINATION OF THE MOTHER (UP TO 6 WEEKS)**

E3 **RESPOND TO OBSERVED SIGNS OR VOLUNTEERED PROBLEMS (1)**
If elevated diastolic pressure

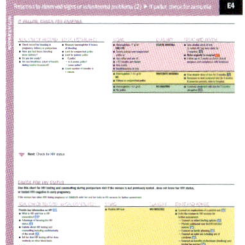

E4 **RESPOND TO OBSERVED SIGNS OR VOLUNTEERED PROBLEMS (2)**
If pallor, check for anaemia

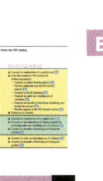

E5 **RESPOND TO OBSERVED SIGNS OR VOLUNTEERED PROBLEMS (3)**
Check for HIV status

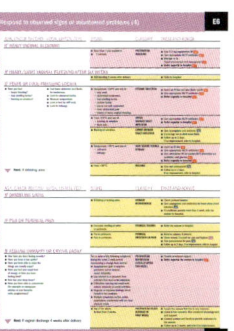

E6 **RESPOND TO OBSERVED SIGNS OR VOLUNTEERED PROBLEMS (4)**
If heavy vaginal bleeding
If fever or foul-smelling lochia

E7 **RESPOND TO OBSERVED SIGNS OR VOLUNTEERED PROBLEMS (5)**
If dribbling urine
If puss or perineal pain
If feeling unhappy or crying easily

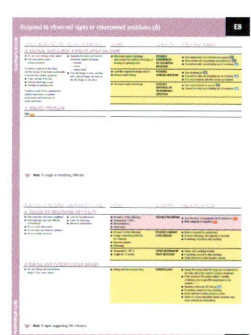

E8 **RESPOND TO OBSERVED SIGNS OR VOLUNTEERED PROBLEMS (6)**
If vaginal discharge 4 weeks after delivery
If breast problem **J9**

E9 **RESPOND TO OBSERVED SIGNS OR VOLUNTEERED PROBLEMS (7)**
If cough or breathing difficulty
If taking anti-tuberculosis drugs

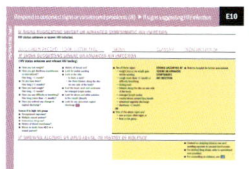

E10 **RESPOND TO OBSERVED SIGNS OR VOLUNTEERED PROBLEMS (8)**
If signs suggesting severe or advanced symptomatic HIV infection

- Always begin with Rapid assessment and management (RAM) **B2-B7**.
- Next use the Postpartum examination of the mother **E2**.
- If an abnormal sign is identified (volunteered or observed), use the charts Respond to observed signs or volunteered problems **E3-E10**.
- Record all treatment given, positive findings, and the scheduled next visit in the home-based and clinic recording form.
- For the first or second postpartum visit during the first week after delivery, use the Postpartum examination chart **D21** and Advise and counselling section **D26** to examine and advise the mother.
- If the woman is HIV-infected, adolescent or has special needs, use **G1-G11** **H1-H4**.

Postpartum care

E1

Postpartum care

To examine the baby see J2-J8.
If breast problem see J9.

E2

POSTPARTUM EXAMINATION OF THE MOTHER (UP TO 6 WEEKS)

Use this chart for examining the mother after discharge from a facility or after home delivery. Record findings in home-based record.
If she delivered less than a week ago without a skilled attendant, use the chart Assess the mother after delivery D21.

ASK, CHECK RECORD

- When and where did you deliver?
- How are you feeling?
- Have you had any pain or fever or bleeding since delivery?
- Do you have any problem with passing urine?
- Ask if the woman has started having sex with her partner.
- Have you decided on any contraception?
- How do your breasts feel?
- Do you have any other concerns?
- Check records:
  → Any complications during delivery?
  → Receiving any treatments?
  → HIV status.
- Ask about tobacco use and exposure to second-hand smoke.

LOOK, LISTEN, FEEL

- Measure blood pressure and temperature.
- Feel uterus. Is it hard and round?
- Look at vulva and perineum for:
  → tear
  → swelling
  → pus.
- Look at pad for bleeding and lochia.
  → Does it smell?
  → Is it profuse?
- Look for pallor.

SIGNS

- Mother feeling well.
- Did not bleed >250 ml.
- Uterus well contracted and hard.
- No perineal swelling.
- Blood pressure, pulse and temperature normal.
- No pallor.
- No breast problem.
- No fever or pain or concern.
- No problem with urination.

CLASSIFY

NORMAL POSTPARTUM

TREAT AND ADVISE

- Make sure woman and family know what to watch for and when to seek care D28.
- Advise on Postpartum care and hygiene, and counsel on nutrition D26.
- Reinforce counselling on safer sexual practices.
- Counsel on the importance of birth spacing and family planning D27.
  Refer for family planning counselling.
- Dispense 3 months iron supply and counsel on compliance F3.
- Give any treatment or prophylaxis due:
  → tetanus immunization if she has not had full course F2.
- Promote use of impregnated bednet for the mother and the baby (or babies).
- Record on the mother's home-based maternal record.
- Advise on when to return to the health facility for the next visit.
- Advise to avoid use of tobacco, alcohol, drugs; and exposure to second-hand smoke.

Next: Respond to observed signs or volunteered problems

RESPOND TO OBSERVED SIGNS OR VOLUNTEERED PROBLEMS

ASK, CHECK RECORD	LOOK, LISTEN, FEEL	SIGNS	CLASSIFY	TREAT AND ADVISE
IF ELEVATED DIASTOLIC BLOOD PRESSURE				
■ History of pre-eclampsia or eclampsia in pregnancy, delivery or after delivery?	■ If diastolic blood pressure is ≥90 mmHg, repeat after a 1 hour rest.	■ Diastolic blood pressure ≥110 mmHg.	**SEVERE HYPERTENSION**	■ Give appropriate antihypertensive B14. ■ **Refer urgently to hospital** B17.
		■ Diastolic blood pressure ≥90 mmHg on 2 readings.	**MODERATE HYPERTENSION**	■ Reassess in 1 week. If hypertension persists, refer to hospital.
		■ Diastolic blood pressure <90 mmHg after 2 readings.	**BLOOD PRESSURE NORMAL**	■ No additional treatment.

▼ **Next:** If pallor, check for anaemia

Respond to observed signs or volunteered problems (1) ▶ **If elevated diastolic blood pressure**

E3

Respond to observed signs or volunteered problems (2) ▶ If pallor, check for anaemia

E4

IF PALLOR, CHECK FOR ANAEMIA

ASK, CHECK RECORD
- Check record for bleeding in pregnancy, delivery or postpartum.
- Have you had heavy bleeding since delivery?
- Do you tire easily?
- Are you breathless (short of breath) during routine housework?

LOOK, LISTEN, FEEL
- Measure haemoglobin if history of bleeding.
- Look for conjunctival pallor.
- Look for palmar pallor.
- If pallor:
  → is it severe pallor?
  → some pallor?
- Count number of breaths in 1 minute.

SIGNS	CLASSIFY	TREAT AND ADVISE
■ Haemoglobin <7 g/dl **AND/OR** ■ Severe palmar and conjunctival pallor or ■ Any pallor and any of: ■ >30 breaths per minute ■ tires easily ■ breathlessness at rest.	**SEVERE ANAEMIA**	■ Give double dose of iron (1 tablet 60 mg twice daily for 3 months) **F3**. ■ **Refer urgently to hospital B17**. ■ Follow up in 2 weeks to check clinical progress and compliance with treatment.
■ Haemoglobin 7-11 g/dl **OR** ■ Palmar or conjunctival pallor.	**MODERATE ANAEMIA**	■ Give double dose of iron for 3 months **F3**. ■ Reassess at next postnatal visit (in 4 weeks). If anaemia persists, refer to hospital.
■ Haemoglobin >11 g/dl. ■ No pallor.	**NO ANAEMIA**	■ Continue treatment with iron for 3 months altogether **F3**.

Next: Check for HIV status

CHECK FOR HIV STATUS

Use this chart for HIV testing and counselling during postpartum visit if the woman is not previously tested, does not know her HIV status, or tested HIV-negative in early pregnancy.

If the woman has taken ARV during pregnancy or childbirth refer her and her baby to HIV services for further assessment.

ASK, CHECK RECORD	LOOK, LISTEN, FEEL	SIGNS	CLASSIFY	TREAT AND ADVISE
Provide key information on HIV G2. ■ What is HIV and how is HIV transmitted G2? ■ Advantage of knowing the HIV status G2. ■ Explain about HIV testing and counselling including confidentiality of the result G3. ■ Tell her that HIV testing will be done routinely as other blood tests. **Ask the woman:** ■ Have you been tested for HIV? → If not: tell her that she will be tested for HIV, unless she refuses. → If yes: check result. → Are you taking any ARV treatment? → Check treatment plan. ■ Has the partner been tested?	■ Perform the Rapid HIV test if not performed in this pregnancy L6.	■ Positive HIV test	**HIV-INFECTED**	■ Counsel on implications of a positive test G3. ■ Refer the woman to HIV services for further assessment and treatment initiation. → Counsel on infant feeding options G7. → Provide additional care for HIV-infected woman G4. → Counsel on family planning G4. → Counsel on safer sex including use of condoms G2. → Counsel on benefits of disclosure (involving) and testing her partner G3. → Provide support to the HIV-infected woman G5. ■ Follow up in 2 weeks.
		■ Negative HIV test	**HIV-NEGATIVE**	■ Counsel on implications of a negative test G3. ■ Counsel on the importance of staying negative by practising safer sex, including use of condoms G2. ■ Counsel on benefits of involving and testing the partner G3.
		■ She refuses the test or is not willing to disclose the result of previous test or no test results available	**UNKNOWN HIV STATUS**	■ Counsel on safer sex including use of condoms G2. ■ Counsel on benefits of involving and testing the partner G3.

 Next: If heavy vaginal bleeding

Respond to observed signs or volunteered problems (4)

E6

POSTPARTUM CARE

ASK, CHECK RECORD LOOK, LISTEN, FEEL	SIGNS	CLASSIFY	TREAT AND ADVISE
IF HEAVY VAGINAL BLEEDING			
	■ More than 1 pad soaked in 5 minutes.	POSTPARTUM BLEEDING	■ Give 0.2 mg ergometrine IM B10. ■ Give appropriate IM/IV antibiotics B15. ■ Manage as in *Rapid assessment and management* B5. ■ **Refer urgently to hospital** B17.
IF HEAVY/LIGHT VAGINAL BLEEDING AFTER SIX WEEKS			
	■ Still bleeding 6 weeks after delivery		■ Refer to hospital
IF FEVER OR FOUL-SMELLING LOCHIA			
■ Have you had: → heavy bleeding? → foul-smelling lochia? → burning on urination? ■ Feel lower abdomen and flanks for tenderness. ■ Look for abnormal lochia. ■ Measure temperature. ■ Look or feel for stiff neck. ■ Look for lethargy.	■ Temperature >38°C and any of: → very weak → abdominal tenderness → foul-smelling lochia → profuse lochia → uterus not well contracted → lower abdominal pain → history of heavy vaginal bleeding.	UTERINE INFECTION	■ Insert an IV line and give fluids rapidly B9. ■ Give appropriate IM/IV antibiotics B15. ■ **Refer urgently to hospital** B17.
	■ Fever >38°C and any of: → burning on urination → flank pain.	UPPER URINARY TRACT INFECTION	■ Give appropriate IM/IV antibiotics B15. ■ **Refer urgently to hospital** B17.
	■ Burning on urination.	LOWER URINARY TRACT INFECTION	■ Give appropriate oral antibiotic F5. ■ Encourage her to drink more fluids. ■ Follow up in 2 days. If no improvement, refer to hospital.
	■ Temperature >38°C and any of: → stiff neck → lethargy.	VERY SEVERE FEBRILE DISEASE	■ Insert an IV line B9. ■ Give appropriate IM/IV antibiotics B15. ■ Give artemether IM (or quinine IM if artemether not available) and glucose B16. ■ **Refer urgently to hospital** B17.
	■ Fever >38°C.	MALARIA	■ Give oral antimalarial F4. ■ Follow up in 2 days. If no improvement, refer to hospital.

▼ **Next:** If dribbling urine

ASK, CHECK RECORD LOOK, LISTEN, FEEL	SIGNS	CLASSIFY	TREAT AND ADVISE
IF DRIBBLING URINE			
	■ Dribbling or leaking urine.	**URINARY INCONTINENCE**	■ Check perineal trauma. ■ Give appropriate oral antibiotics for lower urinary tract infection **F5**. ■ If conditions persists more than 1 week, refer the woman to hospital.
IF PUS OR PERINEAL PAIN			
	■ Excessive swelling of vulva or perineum.	**PERINEAL TRAUMA**	■ Refer the woman to hospital.
	■ Pus in perineum. ■ Pain in perineum.	**PERINEAL INFECTION OR PAIN**	■ Remove sutures, if present. ■ Clean wound. Counsel on care and hygiene **D26**. ■ Give paracetamol for pain **F4**. ■ Follow up in 2 days. If no improvement, refer to hospital.
IF FEELING UNHAPPY OR CRYING EASILY			
■ How have you been feeling recently? ■ Have you been in low spirits? ■ Have you been able to enjoy the things you usually enjoy? ■ Have you had your usual level of energy, or have you been feeling tired? ■ How has your sleep been? ■ Have you been able to concentrate (for example on newspaper articles or your favourite radio programmes)?	Two or more of the following symptoms during the same 2 week period representing a change from normal: ■ Inappropriate guilt or negative persistent sad or anxious mood, irritability. ■ Low interest in or pleasure from activities that used to be enjoyable. ■ Difficulties carrying out usual work, school, domestic or social activities. ■ Negative or hopeless feelings about herself or her newborn. ■ Multiple symptoms (aches, pains, palpitations, numbness) with no clear physical cause.	**POSTPARTUM DEPRESSION (USUALLY AFTER TWO WEEKS)**	■ Provide emotional support. ■ **Refer urgently the woman to hospital B7**.
	■ Any of the above, for less than 2 weeks.	**POSTPARTUM BLUES (USUALLY IN FIRST WEEK)**	■ Assure the woman that this is very common. ■ Listen to her concerns. Give emotional encouragement and support. ■ Counsel partner and family to provide assistance to the woman. ■ Follow up in 2 weeks, and refer if no improvement.

▼ **Next:** If vaginal discharge 4 weeks after delivery

Respond to observed signs or volunteered problems (5)

E7

Respond to observed signs or volunteered problems (6)

E8

POSTPARTUM CARE

ASK, CHECK RECORD	LOOK, LISTEN, FEEL	SIGNS	CLASSIFY	TREAT AND ADVISE

IF VAGINAL DISCHARGE 4 WEEKS AFTER DELIVERY

■ Do you have itching at the vulva? ■ Has your partner had a urinary problem? If partner is present in the clinic, ask the woman if she feels comfortable if you ask him similar questions. ■ If yes, ask him if he has: ■ urethral discharge or pus ■ burning on passing urine. If partner could not be approached, explain importance of partner assessment and treatment to avoid reinfection.	■ Separate the labia and look for abnormal vaginal discharge: → amount → colour → odour/smell. ■ If no discharge is seen, examine with a gloved finger and look at the discharge on the glove.	■ Abnormal vaginal discharge, and partner has urethral discharge or burning on passing urine.	**POSSIBLE GONORRHOEA OR CHLAMYDIA INFECTION**	■ Give appropriate oral antibiotics to woman **F5**. ■ Treat partner with appropriate oral antibiotics **F5**. ■ Counsel on safer sex including use of condoms **G2**.
		■ Curd-like vaginal discharge and/or ■ Intense vulval itching.	**POSSIBLE CANDIDA INFECTION**	■ Give clotrimazole **F5**. ■ Counsel on safer sex including use of condoms **G2**. ■ If no improvement, refer the woman to hospital.
		■ Abnormal vaginal discharge.	**POSSIBLE BACTERIAL OR TRICHOMONAS INFECTION**	■ Give metronidazole to woman **F5**. ■ Counsel on safer sex including use of condoms **G2**.

IF BREAST PROBLEM

See **J9**.

▼ **Next:** If cough or breathing difficulty

ASK, CHECK RECORD / LOOK, LISTEN, FEEL	SIGNS	CLASSIFY	TREAT AND ADVISE
IF COUGH OR BREATHING DIFFICULTY			
■ How long have you been coughing? ■ How long have you had difficulty in breathing? ■ Do you have chest pain? ■ Do you have any blood in sputum? ■ Do you smoke tobacco? ■ Look for breathlessness. ■ Listen for wheezing. ■ Measure temperature.	■ At least 2 of the following: ■ Temperature >38°C. ■ Breathlessness. ■ Chest pain.	**POSSIBLE PNEUMONIA**	■ Give first dose of appropriate IM/IV antibiotics `B15`. ■ **Refer urgently to hospital** `B17`.
	■ At least 1 of the following: ■ Cough or breathing difficulty for >3 weeks. ■ Blood in sputum. ■ Wheezing.	**POSSIBLE CHRONIC LUNG DISEASE**	■ Refer to hospital for assessment. ■ If severe wheezing, refer urgently to hospital. ■ If smoking, counsel to stop smoking
	■ Temperature <38°C. ■ Cough for <3 weeks.	**UPPER RESPIRATORY TRACT INFECTION**	■ Advise safe, soothing remedy. ■ If smoking, counsel to stop smoking. ■ Avoid exposure to other people's smoke.
IF TAKING ANTI-TUBERCULOSIS DRUGS			
■ Are you taking anti-tuberculosis drugs? If yes, since when?	■ Taking anti-tuberculosis drug	**TUBERCULOSIS**	■ Assure the woman that the drugs are not harmful to her baby, and of the need to continue treatment. ■ If her sputum is TB-positive within 2 months of delivery, plan to give INH prophylaxis to the newborn `K13`. ■ Offer HIV testing (if not done) `G3`. ■ If smoking, counsel to stop smoking. ■ Avoid exposure to other people's smoke. ■ Advise to screen immediate family members and close contacts for tuberculosis.

 Next: If signs suggesting HIV infection

Respond to observed signs or volunteered problems (7)

E9

Respond to observed signs or volunteered problems (8) ▶ If signs suggesting HIV infection

E10

IF SIGNS SUGGESTING SEVERE OR ADVANCED SYMPTOMATIC HIV INFECTION

HIV status unknown or known HIV-infected.

ASK, CHECK RECORD	LOOK, LISTEN, FEEL	SIGNS	CLASSIFY	TREAT AND ADVISE

IF SIGNS SUGGESTING SEVERE OR ADVANCED HIV INFECTION

(HIV status unknown)

- Have you lost weight?
- Have you got diarrhoea (continuous or intermittent)? How long, >1 month?
- Do you have fever? How long (>1 month)?
- Have you had cough? How long, >1 month?
- Have you any difficulty in breathing? How long (more than >1 month)?
- Have you noticed any change in vaginal discharge?

Assess if in high risk group:
- Occupational exposure?
- Multiple sexual partner?
- Intravenous drug use?
- History of blood transfusion?
- Illness or death from AIDS in a sexual partner?

- History of forced sex?
- Look for visible wasting.
- Look at the skin:
  → Is there a rash?
  → Are there blisters along the ribs on one side of the body?
- Feel the head, neck and underarm for enlarged lymph nodes.
- Look for ulcers and white patches in the mouth (thrush).
- Look for any abnormal vaginal discharge **C9**.

- Two of these signs:
  → weight loss or no weight gain visible wasting
  → cough more than >1 month or difficulty breathing
  → itching rash
  → blisters along the ribs on one side of the body
  → enlarged lymph nodes
  → cracks/ulcers around lips/mouth
  → abnormal vagainla discharge
  → diarrhoea >1 month.
  OR
- One of the above signs and
  → one or more other signs or
  → from a risk group.

STRONG LIKELIHOOD OF SEVERE OR ADVANCED SYMPTOMATIC HIV INFECTION

- Offer HIV testing and counselling (if not done).
- Refer to hospital for further assessment.

IF SMOKING, ALCOHOL OR DRUG ABUSE, OR HISTORY OF VIOLENCE

- Counsel on stopping tobacco use and avoiding exposure to second-hand smoke.
- For alcohol/drug abuse, refer to specialized care providers.
- For counselling on violence, see **H4**.

PREVENTIVE MEASURES AND ADDITIONAL TREATMENTS FOR THE WOMAN

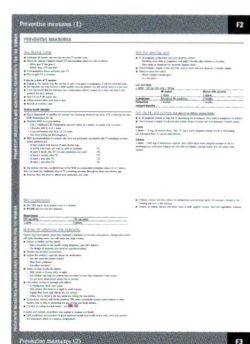

F2 PREVENTIVE MEASURES (1)
Give tetanus toxoid
Give vitamin A postpartum
Give aspirin and calcium

F3 PREVENTIVE MEASURES (2)
Give iron and folic acid
Motivate on compliance with iron treatment
Give mebendazole

F4 ADDITIONAL TREATMENTS FOR THE WOMAN (1)
Give preventive intermittent treatment for falciparum malaria
Advise to use insecticide-treated bednet
Give paracetamol

F5 ADDITIONAL TREATMENTS FOR THE WOMAN (2)
Give appropriate oral antibiotics

F6 ADDITIONAL TREATMENTS FOR THE WOMAN (3)
Give benzathine penicillin IM
Observe for signs of allergy

- This section has details on preventive measures and treatments prescribed in pregnancy and postpartum.
- General principles are found in the section on good practice **A2**.
- For emergency treatment for the woman see **B8-B17**.
- For treatment for the newborn see **K9-K13**.

Preventive measures (1)   F2

PREVENTIVE MEASURES

Give tetanus toxoid

- Immunize all women who are due for their TT vaccine dose
- Check the woman's tetanus toxoid (TT) immunization status by card or history:
  → When was TT last given?
  → Which dose of TT was this?
- If immunization status unknown, give TT1.
- Plan to give TT2 in 4 weeks.

If due for a dose of TT vaccine:

- Explain to the woman that the vaccine is safe to be given in pregnancy; it will not harm the baby.
- The injection site may become a little swollen, red and painful, but this will go away in a few days.
- If she has heard that the injection has contraceptive effects, assure her it does not, that it only protects her from disease.
- Give 0.5 ml TT IM, upper arm.
- Advise woman when next dose is due.
- Record on mother's card.

Tetanus toxoid schedule

- This is dependent on whether the woman has previously received any dose of TT-containing vaccines (DTP/Pentavalent, DT, Td)
- Standard WHO recommendation
  → First 3 childhood DTP/Pentavalent vaccines series at 6 weeks, 10 weeks and 14 weeks.
  → A booster with Td at 4-7 years
  → A second booster with Td at 12-15 years
  → One dose during the first pregnancy
- WHO recommendation for women who were not previously vaccinated with TT-containing vaccines before adolescence
  → At first contact with woman of reproductive age or at first antenatal care visit, as early as possible.   TT1
  → At least 4 weeks after TT1 (at next antenatal care visit).   TT2
  → At least 6 months after TT2.   TT3
  → At least 1 year after TT3.   TT4
  → At least 1 year after TT4.   TT5
- Any woman who has completed any of the WHO recommended schedules above (6 or 5 doses) does not need any additional dose of TT-containing vaccines throughout their reproductive age.

Give iron and folic acid

- To all pregnant, postpartum and post-abortion women:
  → Routinely once daily in pregnancy and until 3 months after delivery or abortion.
  → Twice daily as treatment for anaemia (double dose).
- Check woman's supply of iron and folic acid at each visit and dispense 3 months supply.
- Advise to store iron safely:
  → Where children cannot get it
  → In a dry place.

Iron and folate
1 tablet = 60 mg, folic acid = 400µg

	All women	Women with anaemia
	1 tablet	2 tablets
In pregnancy	Throughout the pregnancy	3 months
Postpartum and post-abortion	3 months	3 months

Give aspirin and calcium (if in area of low dietary calcium intake)

- To all pregnant women at high risk of developing pre-eclampsia. Once daily in pregnancy to delivery
- Check woman's supply of calcium and aspirin tablets at each visit and dispense 3 month supply

Aspirin
1 tablet = 75 mg (or nearest dose). Give 75 mg to every pregnant woman at risk of developing pre-eclampsia from 12 weeks until delivery.

Calcium
1 tablet = 1500 mg of elementary calcium. Give 1500 mg to every pregnant woman at risk of developing pre-eclampsia living in an area with low dietary calcium intake from 20 weeks until delivery.

Give mebendazole

- Give 500 mg to every woman once in 6 months.
- **DO NOT** give it in the first trimester.

Mebendazole

500 mg tablet	100 mg tablet
1 tablet	5 tablets

Motivate on adherence with treatments

Explore local perceptions about iron treatment (examples of incorrect perceptions: making more blood will make bleeding worse, iron will cause too large a baby).

- Explain to mother and her family:
  → Iron is essential for her health during pregnancy and after delivery
  → The danger of anaemia and need for supplementation.
- Discuss any incorrect perceptions.
- Explore the mother's concerns about the medication:
  → Has she used the tablets before?
  → Were there problems?
  → Any other concerns?
- Advise on how to take the tablets
  → With meals or, if once daily, at night
  → Iron tablets may help the patient feel less tired. Do not stop treatment if this occurs
  → Do not worry about black stools. This is normal.
- Give advice on how to manage side-effects:
  → If constipated, drink more water
  → Take tablets after food or at night to avoid nausea
  → Explain that these side effects are not serious
  → Advise her to return if she has problems taking the iron tablets.
- If necessary, discuss with family member, TBA, other community-based health workers or other women, how to help in promoting the use of iron and folate tablets.
- Counsel on eating iron-rich foods – see C16, D26.

If aspirin and calcium prescribed, also explain to woman and family:
- Both medicines are essential for good maternal health and health of the baby, since they prevent pre-eclampsia, which is a serious complication.
- If taking calcium and iron, advise on taking them several hours apart, for example, calcium in the morning and iron in the evening.
- Counsel on eating calcium rich foods, such as milk, yoghurt, cheese, dark leaf vegetables, soybean.

Preventive measures (2)

Additional treatments for the woman (1) ▶ Antimalarial treatment and paracetamol   F4

ANTIMALARIAL TREATMENT AND PARACETAMOL

Give preventive intermittent treatment of falciparum malaria in pregnancy

- Give sulfadoxine-pyrimethamine at antenatal care visits in the second and third trimester to all women according to national policy.
- Check when last dose of sulfadoxine-pyrimethamine given:
  → If no dose in last month, give sulfadoxine-pyrimethamine, 3 tablets in clinic (directly observed therapy - DOT).
- It can be taken on an empty stomach or with food.
- Advise woman when next dose is due.
- Monitor the baby for jaundice if given just before delivery.
- Record on home-based record.

DO NOT give Sulfadoxine+ pyrimethamine to HIV-infected pregnant woman receiving cotrimoxazole prophylaxis.

Sulfadoxine + pyrimethamine
1 tablet = 500 mg sulfadoxine + 25 mg pyrimethamine

	Second trimester		Third trimester	
Month of pregnancy	4	6	8	9
	3 tablets	3 tablets	3 tablets	3 tablets

Advise to use insecticide-treated bednet

- Ask whether woman and newborn will be sleeping under a bednet.
- If yes,
  → Has it been dipped in insecticide?
  → When?
  → Advise to dip every 6 months.
- If not, advise to use insecticide-treated bednet, and provide information to help her do this.

Give appropriate oral antimalarial treatment
(uncomplicated P. falciparum malaria)

A highly effective antimalarial (even if second-line) is preferred during pregnancy

Pregnant woman 1st trimester	Quinine plus clindamycin Tablet 300 mg + capsule 150 mg Give 2 tablets + 2 capsules Every 8 hours + every 6 hours With a glass of water For 7 days OR Quinine monotherapy if clindamycin is not available.	OR	Artesunate plus clindamycin Tablet 50 mg + capsule 150 mg Give 1 tablet + 2 capsules Every 12 hours + every 6 hours For 7 days
2nd and 3rd trimester	Artemisinin-based combined therapy known to be effective in country/region	OR	Artesunate plus clindamycin Tablet 50 mg + capsule 150 mg Give 1 tablet + 2 capsules Every 12 hours + every 6 hours For 7 days OR Quinine plus clindamycin For 7 days
Lactating women	Standard antimalarial therapy, including ACT known to be effective in country/region but not dapsone, primaquine or tetracycline		

If HIV infected and taking zidovudione or efavirenz, if possible, avoid amodiaquine-containing ACT regimens.

Give paracetamol

If severe pain

Paracetamol	Dose	Frequency
1 tablet = 500 mg	1-2 tablets	every 4-6 hours

GIVE APPROPRIATE ORAL ANTIBIOTICS

INDICATION	ANTIBIOTIC	DOSE	FREQUENCY	DURATION	COMMENT
Mastitis	**CLOXACILLIN** 1 capsule (500 mg)	500 mg	every 6 hours	10 days	
Lower urinary tract infection	**AMOXYCILLIN** 1 tablet (500 mg) OR	500 mg	every 8 hours	3 days	
	TRIMETHOPRIM+ SULPHAMETHOXAZOLE 1 tablet (80 mg + 400 mg)	80 mg trimethoprim + 400 mg sulphamethoxazole	two tablets every 12 hours	3 days	Avoid in late pregnancy and two weeks after delivery when breastfeeding.
Gonorrhoea Woman	**CEFTRIAXONE** (Vial=250 mg)	250 mg IM injection	once only	once only	
Partner only	**CIPROFLOXACIN** (1 tablet=250 mg)	500 mg (2 tablets)	once only	once only	Not safe for pregnant or lactating women.
Chlamydia Woman	**ERYTHROMYCIN** (1 tablet=250 mg)	500 mg (2 tablets)	every 6 hours	7 days	
Partner only	**TETRACYCLINE** (1 tablet=250 mg) OR	500 mg (2 tablets)	every 6 hours	7 days	Not safe for pregnant or lactating woman.
	DOXYCYCLINE (1 tablet=100 mg)	100 mg	every 12 hours	7 days	
Trichomonas or bacterial vaginal infection	**METRONIDAZOLE** (1 tablet=500 mg)	2 g or 500 mg	once only every 12 hours	once only 7 days	Do not use in the first trimester of pregnancy.
Vaginal candida infection	**CLOTRIMAZOLE** 1 pessary 200 mg or 500 mg	200 mg 500 mg	every night once only	3 days once only	Teach the woman how to insert a pessary into vagina and to wash hands before and after each application.

Additional treatments for the woman (2) ▶ **Give appropriate oral antibiotics**

Additional treatments for the woman (3) ▶ Give benzathine penicillin IM

F6

GIVE BENZATHINE PENICILLIN IM

Treat the partner. Rule out history of allergy to antibiotics.

INDICATION	ANTIBIOTIC	DOSE	FREQUENCY	DURATION	COMMENT
Syphilis RPR test positive	BENZATHINE PENICILLIN IM (2.4 million units in 5 ml)	2.4 million units IM injection	once only	once only	Give as two IM injections at separate sites. Plan to treat newborn K12. Counsel on correct and consistent use of condoms G2.
If woman has allergy to penicillin	ERYTHROMYCIN (1 tablet = 250 mg)	500 mg (2 tablets)	every 6 hours	15 days	
If partner has allergy to penicillin	TETRACYCLINE (1 tablet = 250 mg) OR DOXYCYCLINE (1 tablet = 100 mg)	500 mg (2 tablets) 100 mg	every 6 hours every 12 hours	15 days 15 days	Not safe for pregnant or lactating woman.

OBSERVE FOR SIGNS OF ALLERGY

After giving penicillin injection, keep the woman for a few minutes and observe for signs of allergy.

ASK, CHECK RECORD	LOOK, LISTEN, FEEL	SIGNS	CLASSIFY	TREAT
■ How are you feeling? ■ Do you feel tightness in the chest and throat? ■ Do you feel dizzy and confused?	■ Look at the face, neck and tongue for swelling. ■ Look at the skin for rash or hives. ■ Look at the injection site for swelling and redness. ■ Look for difficult breathing. ■ Listen for wheezing.	Any of these signs: ■ Tightness in the chest and throat. ■ Feeling dizzy and confused. ■ Swelling of the face, neck and tongue. ■ Injection site swollen and red. ■ Rash or hives. ■ Difficult breathing or wheezing.	**ALLERGY TO PENICILLIN**	■ Open the airway B9. ■ Insert IV line and give fluids B9. ■ Give 0.5 ml adrenaline 1:1000 in 10 ml saline solution IV slowly. Repeat in 5-15 minutes, if required. ■ DO NOT leave the woman on her own. ■ **Refer urgently to hospital** B17.

PREVENTIVE MEASURES AND ADDITIONAL TREATMENTS FOR THE WOMAN

INFORM AND COUNSEL ON HIV

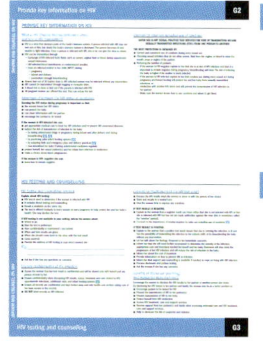

G2 PROVIDE KEY INFORMATION ON HIV
What is HIV and how is HIV transmitted?
Advantage of knowing the HIV status
in pregnancy
Counsel on safer sex including use of condom

G3 HIV TESTING AND COUNSELLING
HIV testing and counselling
Discuss confidentiality of HIV infection
Counsel on implications of the HIV test result
Benefits of disclosure (involving) and testing the male partner(s)

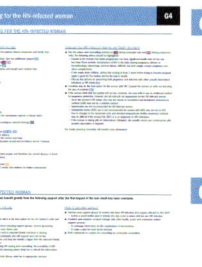

G4 CARE AND COUNSELLING FOR THE HIV-INFECTED WOMAN
Additional care for the HIV-infected woman
Counsel the HIV-infected woman on family planning

G5 SUPPORT TO THE HIV-INFECTED WOMAN
Provide emotional support to the woman
How to provide support

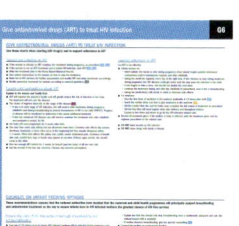

G6 GIVE ANTIRETROVIRAL MEDICINE (ART) TO TREAT HIV INFECTION
Support the initiation of ARV
Support adherence to ARV

G7 COUNSEL ON INFANT FEEDING OPTIONS
Explain the risks of HIV transmission through breastfeeding and not breastfeeding
If a woman does not know her HIV status
If a woman knows that she is HIV-infected

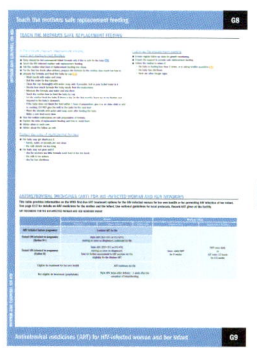

G8 TEACH THE MOTHER SAFE REPLACEMENT FEEDING
If mother chooses replacement feeding:
Teach her replacement feeding.
Explain the risks of replacement feeding
Follow-up for replacement feeding

G9 ANTIRETROVIRAL MEDICINE (ART) TO HIV-INFECTED WOMAN AND HER NEWBORN

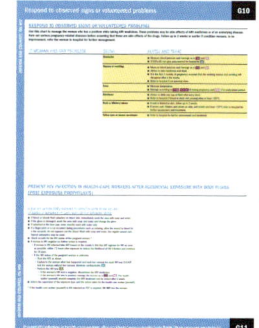

G10 RESPOND TO OBSERVED SIGNS AND VOLUNTEERED PROBLEMS
If a woman is taking antiretroviral medicines and develops new signs/symptoms, respond to her problems

G11 PREVENT HIV INFECTION IN HEALTH-CARE WORKERS AFTER ACCIDENTAL EXPOSURE WITH BODY FLUIDS (POST EXPOSURE PROPHYLAXIS)
If a health-care worker is exposed to body fluids by cuts/pricks/splashes, give him/her appropriate care

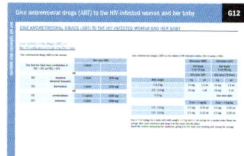

G12 ANTIRETROVIRAL MEDICINES (ART) FOR HIV-INFECTED WOMAN AND HER INFANT ART
Regimens for the HIV-infected woman and her newborn infant
Give antiretroviral medicines (ART) to the woman
Give antiretroviral medicines (ART) to the infant of
HIV-infected mother (first 6 weeks of life)

- Use this section when accurate information on HIV must be given to the woman and her family.

- Provide key information on HIV to all women and explain at the first antenatal care visit how HIV transmitted and the advantages of knowing the HIV status in pregnancy **G2**.

- Explain about HIV testing and counselling, the implications of the test result and benefits of involving and testing the male partner(s). Discuss confidentiality of HIV infection **G3**.

- If the woman is HIV-infected:

- provide additional care during pregnancy, childbirth and postpartum **G4**.

- give any particular support that she may require **G5**.

- Offer antiretroviral treatment **G6**, **G9**.

- Counsel the woman on infant feeding options **G7**.

- Support the mothers choice of infant feeding **G8**.

- Counsel all women on safer sex including use of condoms during and after pregnancy **G2**.

- If the woman taking antiretroviral treatment is having complaints, respond to her problems **G10**.

- If the health-care worker is accidentally exposed to HIV infection, give her/him appropriate care **G11**.

Inform and counsel on HIV

Provide key information on HIV

PROVIDE KEY INFORMATION ON HIV

What is HIV (human immunodeficiency virus) and how is HIV transmitted?

- HIV is a virus that destroys parts of the body's immune system. A person infected with HIV may not feel sick at first, but slowly the body's immune system is destroyed. The person becomes ill and unable to fight infection. Once a person is infected with HIV, she or he can give the virus to others.
- HIV can be transmitted through:
  → Exchange of HIV-infected body fluids such as semen, vaginal fluid or blood during unprotected sexual intercourse.
  → HIV-infected blood transfusions or contaminated needles.
  → From an infected mother to her child (MTCT) during:
    → pregnancy
    → labour and delivery
    → postpartum through breastfeeding.
- Almost four out of 20 babies born to HIV infected women may be infected without any intervention.
- HIV cannot be transmitted through hugging or mosquito bites.
- A blood test is done to find out if the person is infected with HIV.
- All pregnant women are offered this test. They can refuse the test.

Advantage of knowing the HIV status in pregnancy

Knowing the HIV status during pregnancy is important so that:
- the woman knows her HIV status
- can protect her baby
- can share information with her partner
- encourage her partner to be tested

If the woman is HIV-infected she can:
- get appropriate medical care to treat her HIV infection and/or prevent HIV-associated illnesses.
- reduce the risk of transmission of infection to the baby:
  → by taking antiretroviral drugs in pregnancy, during labour and after delivery and during breastfeeding **G6**, **G9**
  → by practicing safer infant feeding options **G9**
  → by adapting birth and emergency plan and delivery practices **G4**.
  → Can breastfeed her baby if taking antiretroviral medicines regularly
- protect herself, her sexual partner(s) and her infant from infection or reinfection.
- make a choice about future pregnancies.

If the woman is HIV- negative she can:
- learn how to remain negative

Counsel on safer sex including use of condoms

SAFER SEX IS ANY SEXUAL PRACTICE THAT REDUCES THE RISK OF TRANSMITTING HIV AND SEXUALLY TRANSMITTED INFECTIONS (STIS) FROM ONE PERSON TO ANOTHER

THE BEST PROTECTION IS OBTAINED BY:
- Correct and consistent use of condoms during every sexual act.
- Choosing sexual activities that do not allow semen, fluid from the vagina, or blood to enter the mouth, anus or vagina of the partner.
- Reducing the number of partners.
  → If the woman is HIV-negative explain to her that she is at risk of HIV infection and that it is important to remain negative during pregnancy, breastfeeding and later. The risk of infecting the baby is higher if the mother is newly infected.
  → If the woman is HIV-infected explain to her that condom use during every sexual act during pregnancy and breast feeding will protect her and her baby from sexually transmitted infections, or
  reinfection with another HIV strain and will prevent the transmission of HIV infection to her partner.
  → Make sure the woman knows how to use condoms and where to get them.

HIV TESTING AND COUNSELLING

HIV testing and Counselling services

Explain about HIV testing:
- HIV test is used to determine if the woman is infected with HIV.
- It includes blood testing and counselling.
- Result is available on the same day.
- The test is offered routinely to every woman at every pregnancy to help protect her and her baby's health. She may decline the test.

If HIV testing is not available in your setting, inform the woman about:
- Where to go.
- How the test is performed.
- How confidentiality is maintained (see below).
- When and how results are given.
- When she should come back to the clinic with the test result
- Costs involved.
- Provide the address of HIV testing in your area's nearest site :

_____
_____

- Ask her if she has any questions or concerns.

Discuss confidentiality of HIV infection

- Assure the woman that her test result is confidential and will be shared only with herself and any person chosen by her.
- Ensure confidentiality when discussing HIV results, status, treatment and care related to HIV, opportunistic infections, additional visits and infant feeding options **A2**.
- Ensure all records are confidential and kept locked away and only health care workers taking care of her have access to the records.
- **DO NOT** label records as HIV-infected.

Counsel on implications of the HIV test result

- Discuss the HIV results when the woman is alone or with the person of her choice.
- State test results in a neutral tone.
- Give the woman time to express any emotions.

IF TEST RESULT IS NEGATIVE:
- Explain to the woman that a negative result can mean either that she is not infected with HIV or that she is infected with HIV but has not yet made antibodies against the virus (this is sometimes called the "window" period).
- Counsel on the importance of staying negative by safer sex including use of condoms **G2**.

IF TEST RESULT IS POSITIVE:
- Explain to the woman that a positive test result means that she is carrying the infection, is ill and has the possibility of transmitting the infection to her unborn child, or by breastfeeding the baby without any intervention.
- Let her talk about her feelings. Respond to her immediate concerns.
- Inform her that she will need further assessment to determine the severity of the infection, appropriate care and treatment needed for herself and her baby. Treatment will slow down the progression of her HIV infection and will reduce the risk of infection to the baby.
- Inform her about the cost of HIV test.
- Provide information on how to prevent HIV re-infection.
- Inform her that support and counselling is available if needed, to cope on living with HIV infection.
- Discuss disclosure and partner testing.
- Ask the woman if she has any concerns.

Benefits of disclosure (involving) and testing the male partner(s)

Encourage the women to disclose the HIV results to her partner or another person she trusts.
By disclosing her HIV status to her partner and family, the woman may be in a better position to:
- Encourage partner to be tested for HIV.
- Prevent the transmission of HIV to her partner(s).
- Prevent transmission of HIV to her baby.
- Protect herself from HIV reinfection.
- Access HIV treatment, care and support services.
- Receive support from her partner(s) and family when accessing antenatal care and HIV treatment, care and support services.
- Help to decrease the risk of suspicion and violence.

Care and counselling for the HIV-infected woman

G4

CARE AND COUNSELLING FOR THE HIV-INFECTED WOMAN

Additional care for the HIV-infected woman

- Determine how much the woman has told her partner, labour companion and family, then respect this confidentiality.
- Be sensitive to her special concerns and fears. Give her additional support `G5`.
- Advise on the importance of good nutrition `C13` `D26`.
- Use standard precautions as for all women `A4`.
- Advise her that she is more prone to infections and should seek medical help as soon as possible if she has:
  → fever
  → persistent diarrhoea
  → cold and cough — respiratory infections
  → burning urination
  → vaginal itching/foul-smelling discharge
  → no weight gain
  → skin infections
  → foul-smelling lochia.

DURING PREGNANCY:
- Revise the birth plan `C2` `C13`.
  → Strongly advise her to deliver in a facility.
  → Advise her to go to a facility as soon as her membranes rupture or labour starts.
- Discuss the infant feeding options `G8-G9`.
- Modify preventive treatment for malaria, according to national strategy `F4`.

DURING CHILDBIRTH:
- Give ART as prescribed in her treatment plan `G6` `G9`, `G12`.
- Adhere to standard practice for labour and delivery.
- Respect confidentiality when giving ART to the mother and baby.
- Record all ART given on labour record, postpartum record and on referral record, if woman is referred.

DURING THE POSTPARTUM PERIOD:
- Tell her that lochia can cause infection in other people and therefore she should dispose of blood stained sanitary pads safely (list local options).
- Counsel her on family planning `G4`.
- If not breastfeeding, advise her on breast care `K8`.
- Tell her to visit HIV services with her baby 2 weeks after delivery for further assessment.

Counsel the HIV-infected woman on family planning

- Use the advice and counselling sections on `C16` during antenatal care and `D27` during postpartum visits. The following advice should be highlighted:
  → Explain to the woman that future pregnancies can have significant health risks for her and her baby. These include: transmission of HIV to the baby (during pregnancy, delivery or breastfeeding), miscarriage, preterm labour, stillbirth, low birth weight, ectopic pregnancy and other complications.
  → If she wants more children, advise that waiting at least 2 years before trying to become pregnant again is good for the mother and for the baby's health.
  → Discuss her options for preventing both pregnancy and infection with other sexually transmitted infections or HIV reinfection.
- Condoms may be the best option for the woman with HIV. Counsel the woman on safer sex including the use of condoms `G2`.
- If the woman thinks that her partner will not use condoms, she may wish to use an additional method for pregnancy protection. However, not all methods are appropriate for the HIV-infected woman:
  → Given the woman's HIV status, she may not choose to breastfeed and lactational amenorrhoea method (LAM) may not be a suitable method.
  → Spermicides are not recommended for HIV-infected women.
  → Intrauterine device (IUD) use is not recommended for women with AIDS who are not on ART.
  → Due to changes in the menstrual cycle and elevated temperatures fertility awareness methods may be difficult if the woman is infected or is on treatment for HIV infections.
  → If the woman is taking pills for tuberculosis (rifampin), she usually cannot use contraceptive pills, monthly injectables or implants.

The family planning counsellor will provide more information.

SUPPORT TO THE HIV-INFECTED WOMAN

Pregnant women who are HIV- infected benefit greatly from the following support after the first impact of the test result has been overcome.

Provide emotional support to the woman

- Empathize with her concerns and fears.
- Use good counselling skills **A2**.
- Help her to assess her situation and decide which is the best option for her, her (unborn) child and her sexual partner. Support her choice.
- Connect her with other existing support services including support groups, income-generating activities, religious support groups, orphan care, home care.
- Help her to find ways to involve her partner and/or extended family members in sharing responsibility, to identify a figure from the community who will support and care for her.
- Discuss how to provide for the other children and help her identify a figure from the extended family or community who will support her children.
- Confirm and support information given during HIV testing and counselling, the possibility of ARV treatment, safe sex, infant feeding and family planning advice (help her to absorb the information and apply it in her own case).
- If the woman has signs of AIDS and/or of other illness, refer her to appropriate services.

How to provide support

- Conduct peer support groups for women who have HIV-infection and couples affected by HIV/AIDS:
  → Led by a social worker and/or woman who has come to terms with her own HIV infection.
- Establish and maintain constant linkages with other health, social and community workers support services:
  → To exchange information for the coordination of interventions
  → To make a plan for each family involved.
- Refer individuals or couples for counselling by community counsellors.

Give antiretroviral drugs (ART) to treat HIV infection　　G6

GIVE ANTIRETROVIRAL DRUGS (ART) TO TREAT HIV INFECTION

Use these charts when starting ARV drug(s) and to support adherence to ART

Support the initiation of ART

- If the woman is already on ART continue the treatment during pregnancy, as prescribed G9, G12.
- If the woman is not on ART treatment and is HIV-infected, start ART G9, G12.
- Write the treatment plan in the Home Based Maternal Record.
- Give written instructions to the woman on how to take the medicines.
- Refer her to HIV services for further assessment and modify ART and other treatments accordingly.
- Modify preventive treatment for malaria according to national guidelines F4.

Discuss importance of ART including benefits and risks

Explain to the woman and family that:
- The evidence shows that early initiation of lifelong ART for both pregnant and breastfeeding women infected with HIV greatly improves women's health and reduces the risk of infection to their babies.
- Her baby will need prophylaxis for 6 weeks after brith.
- She may have some side effects but not all women have them. Common side effects like nausea, diarrhoea, headache or fever often occur in the beginning but they usually disappear within 2–3 weeks. Other side effects like yellow eyes, pallor, severe abdominal pain, shortness of breath, skin rash, painful feet, legs or hands may appear at any time. If these signs persist, she should come to the clinic.
- Give her enough ART tablets for 2 weeks for herself (and her baby) or till her next visit.
- Ask the woman if she has any concerns. Discuss any incorrect perceptions.

Support adherence to ART

For ART to be effective:
- Advise woman on:
  → which tablets she needs to take during pregnancy, labour and after childbirth.
  → taking the medicine regularly, every day, at the right time. If she chooses to stop taking medicines during pregnancy, her HIV disease could get worse and she may pass the infection to her child.
  → if she forgets to take a dose, she should not double the next dose.
  → continue the treatment during and after the childbirth (if prescribed), even if she is breastfeeding.
  → taking the medicine(s) with meals in order to minimize side effects.
- For newborn:
  → Give the first dose of medicine to the newborn preferably 6-12 hours after birth G12.
  → Teach the mother when and how to give treatment to the newborn K13.
  → Tell the mother that she and her baby must complete the full course of treatment as prescribed.
  → Tell her that they will need regular visits after delivery and throughout infancy. Explain to her when and where to go for the HIV-infection related visit.
- Record all treatment given. If the mother or baby is referred, write the treatment given and the regimen prescribed on the referral card.

- **DO NOT** label records as HIV-infected
- **DO NOT** share drugs with family or friends.

INFORM AND COUNSEL ON HIV

COUNSEL ON INFANT FEEDING OPTIONS

These recommendations assume that the national authorities have decided that the maternal and child health programmes will principally support breastfeeding and antiretroviral treatment as the way to ensure infants born to HIV-infected mothers the greatest chance of HIV-free survival.

Explain the risks of HIV transmission through breastfeeding and not breastfeeding

- Four out of 20 babies born to known HIV-infected mothers will be infected during pregnancy and delivery without ART. Three more may be infected by breastfeeding.
- The risk to the infant is very reduced if the mother is receiving ART in pregnancy, during childbirth and during breastfeeding.
- The risk may be reduced if the baby is breastfed exclusively using good technique, so that the breasts stay healthy.
- Mastitis and nipple fissures increase the risk that the baby will be infected.
- The risk of not breastfeeding may be much higher because replacement feeding carries risks too:
  → diarrhoea because of contamination from unclean water, unclean utensils or because the milk is left out too long.
  → malnutrition because of insufficient quantity given to the baby, the milk is too watery, or because of recurrent episodes of diarrhoea.
- Mixed feeding increases the risk of diarrhoea. It may also increase the risk of HIV transmission.

If a woman does not know her HIV status

- Counsel on the importance of exclusive breastfeeding K2.
- Encourage exclusive breastfeeding.
- Counsel on the need to know the HIV status and where to go for HIV testing and counselling G3.
- Explain to her the risks of HIV transmission:
  → even in areas where many women have HIV, most women are negative
  → the risk of infecting the baby is higher if the mother is newly infected
- explain that it is very important to avoid infection during pregnancy and the breastfeeding period.

If a woman knows that she is HIV-infected

- Inform the mother about the most appropriate infant feeding options.
- Counsel the mother on importance of exclusive breastfeeding for her infant.
  → The best for her baby is exclusive breastfeeding for 6 months.
  → At six months baby should begin receiving complementary foods and continue breastfeeding until 12 months old. (Use national guidelines for details.)
  → Tell her that she will be taking ART while breastfeeding.
  → Explain her that she should only stop breastfeeding once a nutritionally adequate and safe diet without breast milk is available.
  → If mother chooses breastfeeding, give her special counselling G7.
- Counsel the mother on replacement feeding.
- Tell her to only give her baby commercial infant formula.
- Assess the conditions needed to safely formula feed:
  → Are safe water and sanitation assured at home and in the community?
  → Is the family able to provide sufficient infant formula milk for baby's needs? K6.
  → Can mother and family members prepare the formula cleanly and frequently enough so that it is safe for the baby?
  → Is family supportive of formula feeding?
  → Does family have access to child health services?
- If the mother chooses replacement feeding teach her to prepare infant formula.
- All babies receiving replacement feeding need regular follow-up, and their mothers need support to provide correct replacement feeding.

Give special counselling to the mother who is HIV-infected and chooses breastfeeding

- Support the mother in her choice of breastfeeding.
- Ensure good attachment and suckling to prevent mastitis and nipple damage K3.
- Advise the mother to return immediately if:
  → she has any breast symptoms or signs
  → the baby has any difficulty feeding.
- Ensure a visit in the first week to assess attachment and positioning and the condition of the mother's breasts.
- Give psychosocial support G5.
- Tell her that if she decides to stop breastfeeding at any time, she must stop gradually within one month. During this time she continues taking ART. Depending to her ART regimen she will either continue taking ART (for life) or will stop ART one week after breastfeeding is fully stopped.
- In some situations an additional possibility is heat-treated expressed breast milk as an interim feeding option if:
  → the baby is born small or ill after birth and temporarily unable to breastfeed;
  → mother is unwell and temporarily unable to breastfeed or has mastitis;
  → antiretroviral drugs are temporarily not available.
  → Teach the mother heat-treating expressed breast milk K5.

Counsel on infant feeding options

G7

Teach the mothers safe replacement feeding

G8

TEACH THE MOTHERS SAFE REPLACEMENT FEEDING

If the mother chooses replacement feeding, teach her replacement feeding

- Baby should be fed commercial infant formula only if this is safe for the baby **G7**.
- Teach the HIV-infected mother safe replacement feeding.
- Ask the mother what kind of replacement feeding she chose.
- For the first few feeds after delivery, prepare the formula for the mother, then teach her how to
- prepare the formula and feed the baby by cup **K9**:
  → Wash hands with water and soap
  → Boil the water for few minutes
  → Clean the cup thoroughly with water, soap and, if possible, boil or pour boiled water in it
  → Decide how much formula the baby needs from the instructions
  → Measure the formula and water and mix them
  → Teach the mother how to feed the baby by cup
  → Let the mother feed the baby 8 times a day (in the first month). Teach her to be flexible and respond to the baby's demands
  → If the baby does not finish the feed within 1 hour of preparation, give it to an older child or add to cooking. DO NOT give the milk to the baby for the next feed
  → Wash the utensils with water and soap soon after feeding the baby
  → Make a new feed every time.
- Give her written instructions on safe preparation of formula.
- Explain the risks of replacement feeding and how to avoid them.
- Advise when to seek care.
- Advise about the follow-up visit.

Explain the risks of replacement feeding

- Her baby may get diarrhoea if:
  → hands, water, or utensils are not clean
  → the milk stands out too long.
- Her baby may not grow well if:
  → she/he receives too little formula each feed or too few feeds
  → the milk is too watery
  → she/he has diarrhoea.

Follow-up for replacement feeding

- Ensure regular follow-up visits for growth monitoring.
- Ensure the support to provide safe replacement feeding.
- Advise the mother to return if:
  → the baby is feeding less than 6 times, or is taking smaller quantities **K6**
  → the baby has diarrhoea
  → there are other danger signs.

INFORM AND COUNSEL ON HIV

ANTIRETROVIRAL MEDICINES (ART) FOR HIV-INFECTED WOMAN AND HER NEWBORN

First-line ART regimens for HIV-infected Pregnant and Breastfeeding Women (for Treatment and Prophylaxis) and Prophylaxis Regimens for HIV-exposed Infants.

	Pregnant and Breastfeeding Women: Regimens for Treatment (Prophylaxis)	HIV-exposed Infants: Regimens for Prophylaxis	
		Breastfeeding	Replacement Feeding
Preferred First Line Regimens	TDF + 3TC (or FTC) + EFV	Once daily NVP for 6 weeks	NVP once daily OR Twice daily AZT For 4-6 weeks
Alternative First-Line Regimens[a,b]	AZT + 3TC + EFV (or NVP) TDF + 3TC (or FTC) + NVP	N/A	N/A
Infant Regimens for Prophylaxis of High Risk[c] Exposure	N/A	Once daily NVP and Twice daily AZT For 6 weeks AND Either NVP alone or NVP/AZT combination for an additional 6 weeks (TOTAL 12 weeks)	Once daily NVP and Twice daily AZT For 6 weeks

a For adults and adolescents d4T should be discontinued as an option in first-line treatment.
b ABC or boosted PIs (ATV/r, DRV/r, LPV/r) can be used in special circumstances.
c High-risk infants are defined as those:
- born to women with established HIV infection who have received less than four weeks of ART at the time of delivery, or
- born to women with established HIV infection with VL >1000 copies/mL in the four weeks before delivery, if VL available, OR
- born to women with incident HIV infection during pregnancy or breastfeeding, OR
- identified for the first time during the postpartum period, with or without a negative HIV test prenatally.

Respond to observed signs or volunteered problems

G10

INFORM AND COUNSEL ON HIV

RESPOND TO OBSERVED SIGNS OR VOLUNTEERED PROBLEMS

Use this chart to manage the woman who has a problem while taking ARV medicines. These problems may be side effects of ARV medicines or of an underlying disease. Rule out serious pregnancy-related diseases before assuming that these are side effects of the drugs. Follow up in 2 weeks or earlier if condition worsens. In no improvement, refer the woman to hospital for further management.

IF WOMAN HAS ANY PROBLEM	SIGNS	ADVISE AND TREAT
	Headache	■ Measure blood pressure and manage as in **C2** and **E3**. ■ If DBP ≤ 90 mm give paracetamol for headache **F4**.
	Nausea or vomiting	■ Measure blood pressure and manage as in **C2** and **E3**. ■ Advise to take medicines with food. ■ If in the first 3 months of pregnancy, reassure that the morning nausea and vomiting will disappear after a few weeks. ■ Refer to hospital if not passing urine.
	Fever	■ Measure temperature. ■ Manage according to **C7-C8**, **C10-C11** if during pregnancy, and **E6-E8** if in postpartum period.
	Diarrhoea	■ Advise to drink one cup of fluid after every stool. ■ Refer to hospital if blood in stool, not passing urine or fever >38°C.
	Rash or blisters/ulcers	■ If rash is limited to skin, follow up in 2 weeks. ■ If severe rash, blisters and ulcers on skin, and mouth and fever >38°C refer to hospital for further assessment and treatment.
	Yellow eyes or mucus membrane	■ Refer to hospital for further assessment and treatment.

PREVENT HIV INFECTION IN HEALTH-CARE WORKERS AFTER ACCIDENTAL EXPOSURE WITH BODY FLUIDS (POST EXPOSURE PROPHYLAXIS)

If you are accidentally exposed to blood or body fluids by cuts or pricks or splashes on face/eyes do the following steps:

- If blood or bloody fluid splashes on intact skin, immediately wash the area with soap and water.
- If the glove is damaged, wash the area with soap and water and change the glove.
- If splashed in the face (eye, nose, mouth) wash with water only.
- If a finger prick or a cut occurred during procedures such as suturing, allow the wound to bleed for a few seconds, do not squeeze out the blood. Wash with soap and water. Use regular wound care. Topical antiseptics may be used.
- Check records for the HIV status of the pregnant woman.*
- If woman is HIV-negative consider repeat testing to confirm negative status shown in records.
  → If woman is HIV-infected take ART based on the country's first line ART regimen for HIV as soon as possible, within 72 hours after exposure to reduce the likelihood of HIV infection and continue for 28 days.
  → If the HIV status of the pregnant woman is unknown:
    → Start the ART as above.
    → Explain to the woman what has happened and seek her consent for rapid HIV test. DO NOT test the woman without her consent. Maintain confidentiality **A2**.
    → Perform the HIV test **L6**.
      → If the woman's HIV test is negative, discontinue the ARV medicines.
      → If the woman's HIV test is positive, manage the woman as in **C2** and **E3**. The health worker (yourself) should complete the ARV treatment and be tested after 6 weeks.
- Inform the supervisor of the exposure type and the action taken for the health-care worker (yourself).

* If the health-care worker (yourself) is HIV-infected no PEP is required. **DO NOT** test the woman.

Give antiretroviral drugs (ART) to the HIV-infected woman and her baby

G12

GIVE ANTIRETROVIRAL DRUGS (ART) TO THE HIV-INFECTED WOMAN AND HER BABY

Give antiretroviral drugs (ART) to the HIV-infected woman and her baby

Give antiretroviral drugs (ART) to the woman

		Give once daily	
Give first-line fixed dose combination of TDF + 3TC (or FTC) + EFV		1 tablet	
OR			
TDF	(tenofovir disoproxil fumarate)	1 tablet	(300 mg)
3TC	(lamivudine)	1 tablet	(300 mg)
OR			
FTC	(emtricitabine)	1 Capsule	(200 mg)
EFV	(efavirenz)	1 tablet	(600 mg)

Give antiretroviral drug(s) (ART) to the HIV-exposed newborn G9 (first 6 weeks of life)

	Nevirapine (NVP)		Zidovudine (AZT)	
	Oral liquid 5 ml=50 mg		Oral liquid 5 ml=50 mg	
	Give once daily		Give every 12 hours	
Birth weight	mg	ml	mg	ml
=>2.5 kg	15 mg	1.5 ml	15 mg	1.5 ml
2.0 - 2.4 kg	10 mg	1 ml	10 mg	1 ml
<2.0 kg				
	Dose = 2 mg/kg		Dose = 2 mg/kg	
1.5 - 1.9 kg	3.5 mg	0.35 ml	3.5 mg	0.35 ml
1.0 - 1.4 kg	2.5 mg	0.25 ml	2.5 mg	0.25 ml

Use a 2 ml syringe for a baby with birth weight =>2 kg and a 1 ml syringe for a smaller baby. Wash the syringe after each treatment and keep it in the clean and dry place.
Teach the mother measuring the medicine, giving it to the baby and cleaning and storing the syringe.

INFORM AND COUNSEL ON HIV

THE WOMAN WITH SPECIAL NEEDS

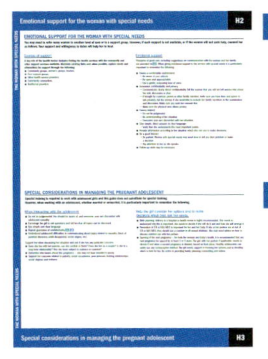

H2 **EMOTIONAL SUPPORT FOR THE WOMAN WITH SPECIAL NEEDS**
Sources of support
Emotional support

H3 **SPECIAL CONSIDERATIONS IN MANAGING THE PREGNANT ADOLESCENT**
When interacting with the adolescent
Help the girl consider her options and to make decisions which best suit her needs

H4 **SPECIAL CONSIDERATIONS FOR SUPPORTING THE WOMAN LIVING WITH VIOLENCE**
Support the woman living with violence
Support the health service response to the needs of women living with violence

- If a woman is an adolescent or living with violence, she needs special consideration. During interaction with such women, use this section to support them.

The woman with special needs   **H1**

Emotional support for the woman with special needs   H2

EMOTIONAL SUPPORT FOR THE WOMAN WITH SPECIAL NEEDS

You may need to refer many women to another level of care or to a support group. However, if such support is not available, or if the woman will not seek help, counsel her as follows. Your support and willingness to listen will help her to heal.

Sources of support

A key role of the health worker includes linking the health services with the community and other support services available. Maintain existing links and, when possible, explore needs and alternatives for support through the following:
- Community groups, women's groups, leaders.
- Peer support groups.
- Other health service providers.
- Community counsellors.
- Traditional providers.

Emotional support

Principles of good care, including suggestions on communication with the woman and her family, are provided on A2 . When giving emotional support to the woman with special needs it is particularly important to remember the following:

- Create a comfortable environment:
    - → Be aware of your attitude
    - → Be open and approachable
    - → Use a gentle, reassuring tone of voice.
- Guarantee confidentiality and privacy:
    - → Communicate clearly about confidentiality. Tell the woman that you will not tell anyone else about the visit, discussion or plan.
    - → If brought by a partner, parent or other family member, make sure you have time and space to talk privately. Ask the woman if she would like to include her family members in the examination and discussion. Make sure you seek her consent first.
    - → Make sure the physical area allows privacy.
- Convey respect:
    - → Do not be judgmental
    - → Be understanding of her situation
    - → Overcome your own discomfort with her situation.
- Give simple, direct answers in clear language:
    - → Verify that she understands the most important points.
- Provide information according to her situation which she can use to make decisions.
- Be a good listener:
    - → Be patient. Women with special needs may need time to tell you their problem or make a decision
    - → Pay attention to her as she speaks.
- Follow-up visits may be necessary.

SPECIAL CONSIDERATIONS IN MANAGING THE PREGNANT ADOLESCENT

Special training is required to work with adolescent girls and this guide does not substitute for special training.
However, when working with an adolescent, whether married or unmarried, it is particularly important to remember the following.

When interacting with the adolescent

- Do not be judgemental. You should be aware of, and overcome, your own discomfort with adolescent sexuality.
- Encourage the girl to ask questions and tell her that all topics can be discussed.
- Use simple and clear language.
- Repeat guarantee of confidentiality `A2` `G3`.
- Understand adolescent difficulties in communicating about topics related to sexuality (fears of parental discovery, adult disapproval, social stigma, etc).

Support her when discussing her situation and ask if she has any particular concerns:
- Does she live with her parents, can she confide in them? Does she live as a couple? Is she in a long-term relationship? Has she been subject to violence or coercion?
- Determine who knows about this pregnancy — she may not have revealed it openly.
- Support her concerns related to puberty, social acceptance, peer pressure, forming relationships, social stigmas and violence.

Help the girl consider her options and to make decisions which best suit her needs.

- Birth planning: delivery in a hospital or health centre is highly recommended. She needs to understand why this is important, she needs to decide if she will do it and and how she will arrange it.
- Prevention of STI or HIV/AIDS is important for her and her baby. If she or her partner are at risk of STI or HIV/AIDS, they should use a condom in all sexual relations. She may need advice on how to discuss condom use with her partner.
- Spacing of the next pregnancy — for both the woman and baby's health, it is recommended that any next pregnancy be spaced by at least 2 or 3 years. The girl, with her partner if applicable, needs to decide if and when a second pregnancy is desired, based on their plans. Healthy adolescents can safely use any contraceptive method. The girl needs support in knowing her options and in deciding which is best for her. Be active in providing family planning counselling and advice.

The woman living with violence

H4

SPECIAL CONSIDERATIONS FOR SUPPORTING THE WOMAN LIVING WITH VIOLENCE

Violence against women by their intimate partners affects women's physical and mental health, including their reproductive health. While you may not have been trained to deal with this problem, women may disclose violence to you or you may see unexplained bruises and other injuries which make you suspect she may be suffering abuse. The following are some recommendations on how to respond and support her.

Support the woman living with violence

- Provide a space where the woman can speak to you in privacy where her partner or others cannot hear. Do all you can to guarantee confidentiality, and reassure her of this.
- Gently encourage her to tell you what is happening to her. You may ask indirect questions to help her tell her story.
- Listen to her in a sympathetic manner. Listening can often be of great support. Do not blame her or make a joke of the situation. She may defend her partner's action. Reassure her that she does not deserve to be abused in any way.
- Help her to assess her present situation. If she thinks she or her children are in danger, explore together the options to ensure her immediate safety (e.g. can she stay with her parents or friends? Does she have, or could she borrow, money?)
- Explore her options with her. Help her identify local sources of support, either within her family, friends, and local community or through NGOs, shelters or social services, if available. Remind her that she has legal recourse, if relevant.
- Offer her an opportunity to see you again. Violence by partners is complex, and she may be unable to resolve her situation quickly.
- Document any forms of abuse identified or concerns you may have in the file.

Support the health service response to needs of women living with violence

- Help raise awareness among health care staff about violence against women and its prevalence in the community the clinic serves.
- Find out what if training is available to improve the support that health care staff can provide to those women who may need it.
- Display posters, leaflets and other information that condemn violence, and information on groups that can provide support.
- Make contact with organizations working to address violence in your area. Identify those that can provide support for women in abusive relationships. If specific services are not available, contact other groups such as churches, women's groups, elders, or other local groups and discuss with them support they can provide or other what roles they can play, like resolving disputes. Ensure you have a list of these resources available.

COMMUNITY SUPPORT FOR MATERNAL AND NEWBORN HEALTH

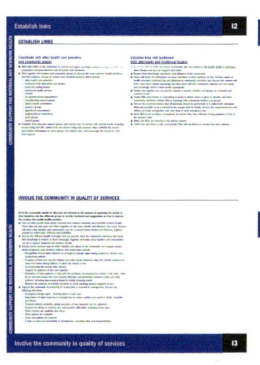

I2 ESTABLISH LINKS
Coordinate with other health care providers and community groups
Establish links with traditional birth attendants and traditional healers

I3 INVOLVE THE COMMUNITY IN QUALITY OF SERVICES

- Everyone in the community should be informed and involved in the process of improving the health of their community members. This section provides guidance on how their involvement can help improve the health of women and newborns.
- Different groups should be asked to give feedback and suggestions on how to improve the services the health facilities provide.
- Use the following suggestions when working with families and communities to support the care of women and newborns during pregnancy, delivery, post-abortion and postpartum periods.

Community support for maternal and newborn health

Establish links

ESTABLISH LINKS

Coordinate with other health care providers and community groups

- Meet with others in the community to discuss and agree messages related to pregnancy, delivery, postpartum and post-abortion care of women and newborns.
- Work together with leaders and community groups to discuss the most common health problems and find solutions. Groups to contact and establish relations which include:
  → other health care providers
  → traditional birth attendants and healers
  → maternity waiting homes
  → adolescent health services
  → schools
  → non-governmental organizations
  → breastfeeding support groups
  → district health committees
  → women's groups
  → agricultural associations
  → neighbourhood committees
  → youth groups
  → church groups.
- Establish links with peer support groups and referral sites for women with special needs, including women living with HIV, adolescents and women living with violence. Have available the names and contact information for these groups and referral sites, and encourage the woman to seek their support.

Establish links with traditional birth attendants and traditional healers

- Contact traditional birth attendants and healers who are working in the health facility's catchment area. Discuss how you can support each other.
- Respect their knowledge, experience and influence in the community.
- Share with them the information you have and listen to their opinions on this. Provide copies of health education materials that you distribute to community members and discuss the content with them. Have them explain knowledge that they share with the community. Together you can create new knowledge which is more locally appropriate.
- Review how together you can provide support to women, families and groups for maternal and newborn health.

- Involve TBAs and healers in counselling sessions in which advice is given to families and other community members. Include TBAs in meetings with community leaders and groups.
- Discuss the recommendation that all deliveries should be performed by a skilled birth attendant. When not possible or not preferred by the woman and her family, discuss the requirements for safer delivery at home, postpartum care, and when to seek emergency care.
- Invite TBAs to act as labour companions for women they have followed during pregnancy, if this is the woman's wish.
- Make sure TBAs are included in the referral system.
- Clarify how and when to refer, and provide TBAs with feedback on women they have referred.
- WHO guidelines for the treatment of malaria. Third edition. April 2015 http://www.who.int/malaria/publications/atoz/9789241549127/en/.
- WHO guidelines on hand hygiene in healthcare (2009). http://apps.who.int/iris/bitstream/10665/44102/1/9789241597906_eng.pdf.
- HO recommendations for prevention and treatment of maternal peripartum infections. 2015. http://www.who.int/reproductivehealth/publications/maternal_perinatal_health/peripartum-infections-guidelines/en/.
- 19th WHO Model List of Essential Medicines (April 2015).
- http://www.who.int/selection_medicines/committees/expert/20/EML_2015_FINAL_amended_AUG2015.pdf?ua=1&ua=1.
- WHO. Safe abortion: technical and policy guidance for health systems. Second edition, 2012. http://www.who.int/reproductivehealth/publications/unsafe_abortion/9789241548434/en/.
- World Health Organization. Consolidated guidelines on the use of antiretroviral drugs for treating and preventing HIV infection: what's new. Policy brief. 2015. http://www.who.int/hiv/pub/arv/policy-brief-arv-2015/en/.
- World Health Organization. Medical eligibility criteria for contraceptive use. Fifth edition, 2015. http://www.who.int/reproductivehealth/publications/family_planning/MEC-5/en/.
- World Health Organization. WHO recommendations on Postnatal care of the mother and newborn. 2013.
- http://www.who.int/maternal_child_adolescent/documents/postnatal-care-recommendations/en/.
- WHO recommendations on interventions to improve preterm birth outcomes. http://www.who.int/reproductivehealth/publications/maternal_perinatal_health/preterm-birth-guideline/en/.
- World Health Organization. Guidelines on basic newborn resuscitation. 2012
- http://www.who.int/maternal_child_adolescent/documents/basic_newborn_resuscitation/en/.
- World Health Organization. Pocket book of hospital care for children: Second edition. Guidelines for the management of common childhood illnesses. 2013. http://www.who.int/maternal_child_adolescent/documents/child_hospital_care/en/.

INVOLVE THE COMMUNITY IN QUALITY OF SERVICES

All in the community should be informed and involved in the process of improving the health of their members. Ask the different groups to provide feedback and suggestions on how to improve the services the health facility provides.

- Find out what people know about maternal and newborn mortality and morbidity in their locality. Share data you may have and reflect together on why these deaths and illnesses may occur. Discuss with them what families and communities can do to prevent these deaths and illnesses. Together prepare an action plan, defining responsibilities.
- Discuss the different health messages that you provide. Have the community members talk about their knowledge in relation to these messages. Together determine what families and communities can do to support maternal and newborn health.
- Discuss some practical ways in which families and others in the community can support women during pregnancy, post-abortion, delivery and postpartum periods:
    - → Recognition of and rapid response to emergency/danger signs during pregnancy, delivery and postpartum periods.
    - → Provision of food and care for children and other family members when the woman needs to be away from home during delivery, or when she needs to rest.
    - → Accompanying the woman after delivery.
    - → Support for payment of fees and supplies.
    - → Motivation of male partners to help with the workload, accompany the woman to the clinic, allow her to rest and ensure she eats properly. Motivate communication between males and their partners, including discussing postpartum family planning needs.
    - → Motivate the partners and family members to avoid smoking around pregnant women.
- Support the community in preparing an action plan to respond to emergencies. Discuss the following with them:
    - → Emergency/danger signs - knowing when to seek care.
    - → Importance of rapid response to emergencies to reduce mother and newborn death, disability and illness.
    - → Transport options available, giving examples of how transport can be organized.
    - → Reasons for delays in seeking care and possible difficulties, including heavy rains.
    - → What services are available and where.
    - → What options are available.
    - → Costs and options for payment.
    - → A plan of action for responding in emergencies, including roles and responsibilities.

NEWBORN CARE

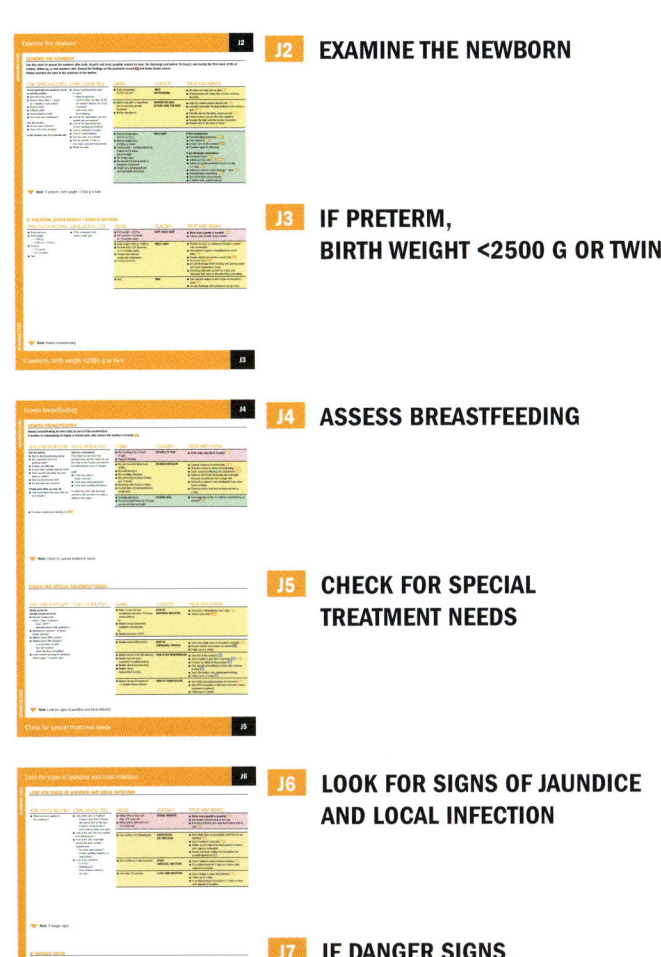

J2 EXAMINE THE NEWBORN

J3 IF PRETERM, BIRTH WEIGHT <2500 G OR TWIN

J4 ASSESS BREASTFEEDING

J5 CHECK FOR SPECIAL TREATMENT NEEDS

J6 LOOK FOR SIGNS OF JAUNDICE AND LOCAL INFECTION

J7 IF DANGER SIGNS

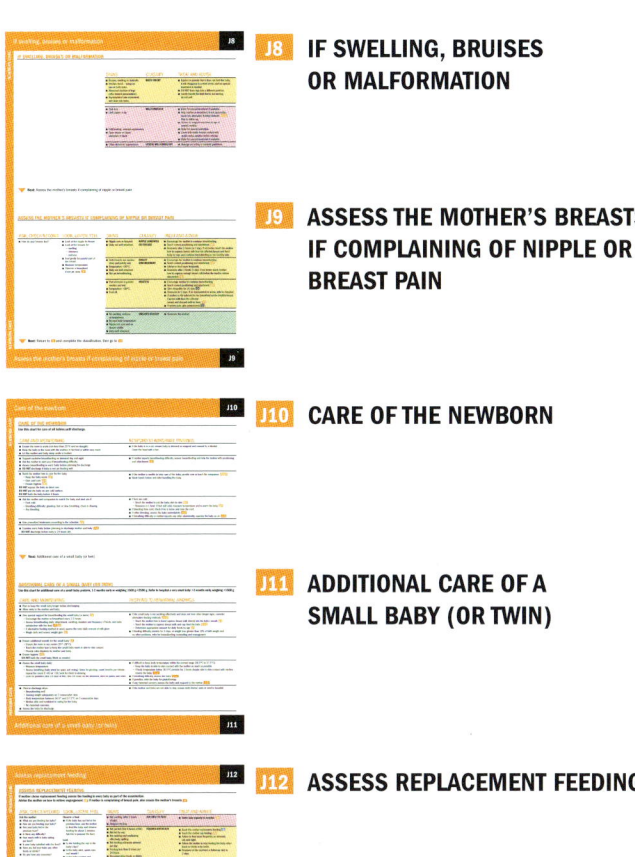

J8 IF SWELLING, BRUISES OR MALFORMATION

J9 ASSESS THE MOTHER'S BREASTS IF COMPLAINING OF NIPPLE OR BREAST PAIN

J10 CARE OF THE NEWBORN

J11 ADDITIONAL CARE OF A SMALL BABY (OR TWIN)

J12 ASSESS REPLACEMENT FEEDING

- Examinine routinely all babies around an hour of birth, for discharge, at routine and follow-up postnatal visits in the first weeks of life, and when the provider or mother observes danger signs.
- Use the chart Assess the mother's breasts if the mother is complaining of nipple or breast pain **J9**.
- During the stay at the facility, use the Care of the newborn chart **J10**. If the baby is small but does not need referral, also use the Additional care for a small baby or twin chart **J11**.
- Use the Breastfeeding, care, preventive measures and treatment for the newborn sections for details of care, resuscitation and treatments **K1-K13**.
- Use Advise on when to return with the baby **K14** for advising the mother when to return with the baby for routine and follow-up visits and to seek care or return if baby has danger signs. Use information and counselling sheets **M5-M6**.
- For care at birth and during the first hours of life, use Labour and delivery **D19**.

ALSO SEE:
- Counsel on choices of infant feeding and HIV-related issues **G7-G8**.
- Equipment, supplies and drugs **L1-L5**.
- Records **N1-N7**.
- Baby dead **D24**.

Newborn care

J1

Examine the newborn

J2

EXAMINE THE NEWBORN

Use this chart to assess the newborn after birth, classify and treat, possibly around an hour; for discharge (not before 24 hours); and during the first week of life at routine, follow-up, or sick newborn visit. Record the findings on the postnatal record **N6** and home-based record.
Always examine the baby in the presence of the mother.

ASK, CHECK RECORD

Check maternal and newborn record or ask the mother:
- How old is the baby?
- Preterm (less than 37 weeks or 1 month or more early)?
- Breech birth?
- Difficult birth?
- Resuscitated at birth?
- Has baby had convulsions?
- Frequent, heavy vomiting?

Ask the mother:
- Do you have concerns?
- How is the baby feeding?

Is the mother very ill or transferred?

LOOK, LISTEN, FEEL

- Assess breathing (baby must be calm)
  → listen for grunting
  → count breaths: are they 30-60 per minute? Repeat the count if elevated
  → look at the chest for in-drawing.
- Look at the movements: are they normal and symmetrical?
- Look at the presenting part — is there swelling and bruises?
- Look at abdomen for pallor and distension.
- Look for malformations.
- Feel the tone: is it normal?
- Feel for warmth. If cold, or very warm, measure temperature.
- Weigh the baby.

SIGNS / CLASSIFY / TREAT AND ADVISE

SIGNS	CLASSIFY	TREAT AND ADVISE
■ Body temperature 35.5°C-36.4°C.	**MILD HYPOTHERMIA**	■ Re-warm the baby skin-to-skin **K9**. ■ If temperature not rising after 2 hours, reassess the baby **J7**.
■ Mother not able to breastfeed due to receiving special treatment. ■ Mother transferred.	**MOTHER NOT ABLE TO TAKE CARE FOR BABY**	■ Help the mother express breast milk **K5**. ■ Consider alternative feeding methods until mother is well **K5-K6**. ■ Provide care for the baby, ensure warmth **K9**. ■ Ensure mother can see the baby regularly. ■ Transfer the baby with the mother if possible. ■ Ensure care for the baby at home.
■ Normal temperature: 36.5°C-37.5°C. ■ Normal weight baby (2500 g or more). ■ Feeding well — suckling effectively 8 times in 24 hours, day and night. ■ No danger signs. ■ No special treatment needs or treatment completed. ■ Small baby, feeding well and gaining weight adequately.	**WELL BABY**	**If first examination:** ■ Breastfeeding counseling **K2-K3**. ■ Give vitamin K **K12**. ■ Ensure care for the newborn **J10**. ■ Examine again for discharge. **If pre-discharge examination:** ■ Immunize if due **K13**. ■ Advise on baby care **K2**, **K9-K10**. ■ Advise on routine postnatal contacts at age 3-7 days **K14**. ■ Advise on when to return if danger signs **K14**. ■ Breastfeeding counselling **K2-K3**. ■ Record in home-based record. ■ If further visits, repeat advices.

▼ **Next:** If preterm, birth weight <2500 g or twin

IF PRETERM, BIRTH WEIGHT <2500-G OR TWIN

ASK, CHECK RECORD
- Baby just born.
- Birth weight
  - → <1500 g
  - → 1500 g to <2500 g.
- Preterm
  - → <32 weeks
  - → 33-36 weeks.
- Twin.

LOOK, LISTEN, FEEL
- If this is repeated visit, assess weight gain

SIGNS	CLASSIFY	TREAT AND ADVISE
■ Birth weight <1500 g. ■ Very preterm <32 weeks or >2 months early).	**VERY SMALL BABY**	■ **Refer baby urgently to hospital** K14. ■ Ensure extra warmth during referral. ■ Ensure appropriate caloric intake K6.
■ Birth weight 1500 g.-<2500 g. ■ Preterm baby (32-36 weeks or 1-2 months early). ■ Several days old and weight gain inadequate. ■ Feeding difficulty.	**SMALL BABY**	■ Provide as close to continuous Kangaroo mother care as possible. ■ Give special support to breastfeed the small baby K4. ■ Ensure appropriate caloric intake. ■ Ensure additional care for a small baby J11. ■ Reassess daily J11. ■ Do not discharge before feeding well, gaining weight and body temperature stable. ■ If feeding difficulties persist for 3 days and otherwise well, refer for breastfeeding counselling.
■ Twin	**TWIN**	■ Give special support to the mother to breastfeed twins K4. ■ Do not discharge until both twins can go home.

▼ **Next:** Assess breastfeeding

If preterm, birth weight <2500-g or twin

J3

Assess breastfeeding J4

ASSESS BREASTFEEDING

Assess breastfeeding in every baby as part of the examination.
If mother is complaining of nipple or breast pain, also assess the mother's breasts **J9**.

ASK, CHECK RECORD

Ask the mother
- How is the breastfeeding going?
- Has your baby fed in the previous hour?
- Is there any difficulty?
- Is your baby satisfied with the feed?
- Have you fed your baby any other foods or drinks?
- How do your breasts feel?
- Do you have any concerns?

If baby more than one day old:
- How many times has your baby fed in 24 hours?

LOOK, LISTEN, FEEL

Observe a breastfeed.
If the baby has not fed in the previous hour, ask the mother to put the baby on her breasts and observe breastfeeding for about 5 minutes.

Look
- Is the baby able to attach correctly?
- Is the baby well-positioned?
- Is the baby suckling effectively?

If mother has fed in the last hour, ask her to tell you when her baby is willing to feed again.

SIGNS	CLASSIFY	TREAT AND ADVISE
■ Not suckling (after 6 hours of age). ■ Stopped feeding.	**NOT ABLE TO FEED**	■ Refer baby urgently to hospital **K14**.
■ Not yet breastfed (first hours of life). ■ Not well attached. ■ Not suckling effectively. ■ Breastfeeding less than 8 times per 24 hours. ■ Receiving other foods or drinks. ■ Several days old and inadequate weight gain.	**FEEDING DIFFICULTY**	■ Support exclusive breastfeeding **K2-K3**. ■ Help the mother to initiate breastfeeding **K3-K4**. ■ Teach correct positioning and attachment **K3-K4**. ■ Advise to feed more frequently, day and night. Reassure her that she has enough milk. ■ Advise the mother to stop feeding the baby other foods or drinks. ■ Reassess at the next feed or follow-up visit in 2 days.
■ Suckling effectively. ■ Breastfeeding 8 times in 24 hours on demand day and night	**FEEDING WELL**	■ Encourage the mother to continue breastfeeding on demand **K3**.

■ To assess replacement feeding see **J12**.

Next: Check for special treatment needs

CHECK FOR SPECIAL TREATMENT NEEDS

ASK, CHECK RECORD   LOOK, LISTEN, FEEL | SIGNS | CLASSIFY | TREAT AND ADVISE

Check record for special treatment needs
- Has the mother had within 2 days of delivery:
  → fever >38°C?
  → infection treated with antibiotics?
- Membranes ruptured >18 hours before delivery?
- Mother tested RPR-positive?
- Mother tested HIV-infected?
  → is or has been on ARV
  → has she received infant feeding counselling?
- Is the mother receiving TB treatment which began <2 months ago?

SIGNS	CLASSIFY	TREAT AND ADVISE
■ Baby <1 day old and membranes ruptured >18 hours before delivery, **or** ■ Mother being treated with antibiotics for infection, **or** ■ Mother has fever >38°C.	**RISK OF BACTERIAL INFECTION**	■ Give baby 2 IM antibiotics for 5 days K12. ■ Assess baby daily J2-J7.
■ Mother tested RPR-positive.	**RISK OF CONGENITAL SYPHILIS**	■ Give baby single dose of benzathine penicillin K12. ■ Ensure mother and partner are treated F6. ■ Follow up in 2 weeks.
■ Mother known to be HIV-infected. ■ Mother has not been counselled on infant feeding. ■ Mother chose breastfeeding. ■ Mother chose replacement feeding.	**RISK OF HIV TRANSMISSION**	■ Give ARV to the newborn G12. ■ Teach mother to give ARV to her baby G12, K13. ■ Counsel on infant feeding options G7. ■ Give special counselling to mother who is breast feeding G7. ■ Teach the mother safe replacement feeding. ■ Follow up in 2 weeks G8.
■ Mother started TB treatment <2 months before delivery.	**RISK OF TUBERCULOSIS**	■ Give baby isoniazid propylaxis for 6 months K13. ■ Give BCG vaccination to the baby only when baby's treatment completed. ■ Follow up in 2 weeks.

 Next: Look for signs of jaundice and local infection

Check for special treatment needs

Look for signs of jaundice and local infection

J6

LOOK FOR SIGNS OF JAUNDICE AND LOCAL INFECTION

ASK, CHECK RECORD	LOOK, LISTEN, FEEL	SIGNS	CLASSIFY	TREAT AND ADVISE
■ What has been applied to the umbilicus?	■ Look at the skin, is it yellow? → if baby is less than 24 hours old, look at skin on the face → if baby is 24 hours old or more, look at palms and soles. ■ Look at the eyes. Are they swollen and draining pus? ■ Look at the skin, especially around the neck, armpits, inguinal area: → Are there skin pustules? → Is there swelling, hardness or large bullae? ■ Look at the umbilicus: → Is it red? → Draining pus? → Does redness extend to the skin?	■ Yellow skin on face and only <24 hours old. ■ Yellow palms and soles and ≥24 hours old.	**SEVERE JAUNDICE**	■ **Refer baby urgently to hospital** K14. ■ Encourage breastfeeding on the way. ■ If feeding difficulty, give expressed breast milk by cup K6.
		■ Eyes swollen and draining pus.	**GONOCOCCAL EYE INFECTION**	■ Give single dose of appropriate antibiotic for eye infection K12. ■ Teach mother to treat eyes K13. ■ Follow up in 2 days. If no improvement or worse, refer urgently to hospital. ■ Assess and treat mother and her partner for possible gonorrhea E8.
		■ Red umbilicus or skin around it.	**LOCAL UMBILICAL INFECTION**	■ Teach mother to treat umbilical infection K13. ■ If no improvement in 2 days, or if worse, refer urgently to hospital.
		■ Less than 10 pustules.	**LOCAL SKIN INFECTION**	■ Teach mother to treat skin infection K13. ■ Follow up in 2 days. ■ If no improvement of pustules in 2 days or more, refer urgently to hospital.

Next: If danger signs

IF DANGER SIGNS

SIGNS	CLASSIFY	TREAT AND ADVISE
Any of the following signs: ■ Fast breathing (more than 60 breaths per minute). ■ Slow breathing or gasping (less than 30 breaths per minute). ■ Severe chest in-drawing. ■ Not feeding well. ■ Grunting. ■ Fits or convulsions ■ Abdominal overdistension ■ Diffuse cyanosis ■ Heart rate constantly > 180/min (cons). ■ Floppy or stiff. ■ No spontaneous movement, floppy or stiff. ■ Temperature >37.5°C. ■ Temperature <35.5°C or not rising after rewarming. ■ Umbilicus draining pus or umbilical redness and swelling extending to skin. ■ More than 10 skin pustules or bullae, or swelling, redness, hardness of skin. ■ Bleeding from stump or cut. ■ Pallor.	**POSSIBLE SERIOUS ILLNESS**	■ Give first dose of 2 IM antibiotics **K12**. ■ **Refer baby urgently to hospital** **K14**. **In addition:** ■ Re-warm and keep warm during referral **K9**. ■ Treat local umbilical infection before referral **K13**. ■ Treat skin infection before referral **K13**. ■ Stop the bleeding.

▼ **Next:** If swelling, bruises or malformation

If swelling, bruises or malformation

J8

IF SWELLING, BRUISES OR MALFORMATION

SIGNS	CLASSIFY	TREAT AND ADVISE
■ Bruises, swelling on buttocks. ■ Swollen head — bump on one or both sides. ■ Abnormal position of legs (after breech presentation). ■ Asymmetrical arm movement, arm does not move.	BIRTH INJURY	■ Explain to parents that it does not hurt the baby, it will disappear in a week or two and no special treatment is needed. ■ DO NOT force legs into a different position. ■ Gently handle the limb that is not moving, do not pull.
■ Club foot ■ Cleft palate or lip	MALFORMATION	■ Refer for special treatment if available. ■ Help mother to breastfeed. If not successful, teach her alternative feeding methods K5-K6. Plan to follow up. ■ Advise on surgical correction at age of several months.
■ Odd looking, unusual appearance ■ Open tissue on head, abdomen back, perineum or genital areas.		■ Refer for special evaluation. ■ Cover with sterile tissues soaked with sterile saline solution before referral. ■ Refer for special treatment if available.
■ Other abnormal appearance.	SEVERE MALFORMATION	■ Manage according to national guidelines.

Next: Assess the mother's breasts if complaining of nipple or breast pain

ASSESS THE MOTHER'S BREASTS IF COMPLAINING OF NIPPLE OR BREAST PAIN

ASK, CHECK RECORD	LOOK, LISTEN, FEEL	SIGNS	CLASSIFY	TREAT AND ADVISE
■ How do your breasts feel?	■ Look at the nipple for fissure ■ Look at the breasts for: → swelling → shininess → redness. ■ Feel gently for painful part of the breast. ■ Measure temperature. ■ Observe a breastfeed if not yet done **J4**.	■ Nipple sore or fissured. ■ Baby not well attached.	**NIPPLE SORENESS OR FISSURE**	■ Encourage the mother to continue breastfeeding. ■ Teach correct positioning and attachment **K3**. ■ Reassess after 2 feeds (or 1 day). If not better, teach the mother how to express breast milk from the affected breast and feed baby by cup, and continue breastfeeding on the healthy side.
		■ Both breasts are swollen, shiny and patchy red. ■ Temperature <38°C. ■ Baby not well attached. ■ Not yet breastfeeding.	**BREAST ENGORGEMENT**	■ Encourage the mother to continue breastfeeding. ■ Teach correct positioning and attachment **K3**. ■ Advise to feed more frequently. ■ Reassess after 2 feeds (1 day). If not better, teach mother how to express enough breast milk before the feed to relieve discomfort **K5**.
		■ Part of breast is painful, swollen and red. ■ Temperature >38°C. ■ Feels ill.	**MASTITIS**	■ Encourage mother to continue breastfeeding. ■ Teach correct positioning and attachment **K3**. ■ Give cloxacillin for 10 days **F5**. ■ Reassess in 2 days. If no improvement or worse, refer to hospital. ■ If mother is HIV-infected let her breastfeed on the healthy breast. Express milk from the affected breast and discard until no fever **K5**. ■ If severe pain, give paracetamol **F4**.
		■ No swelling, redness or tenderness. ■ Normal body temperature. ■ Nipple not sore and no fissure visible. ■ Baby well attached.	**BREASTS HEALTHY**	■ Reassure the mother.

▼ **Next:** Return to **J2** and complete the classification, then go to **J10**.

Assess the mother's breasts if complaining of nipple or breast pain

Care of the newborn J10

CARE OF THE NEWBORN

Use this chart for care of all babies until discharge.

CARE AND MONITORING	RESPOND TO ABNORMAL FINDINGS
■ Ensure the room is warm (not less than 25°C and no draught). ■ Keep the baby in the room with the mother, in her bed or within easy reach. ■ Let the mother and baby sleep under a bednet.	■ If the baby is in a cot, ensure baby is dressed or wrapped and covered by a blanket. Cover the head with a hat.
■ Support exclusive breastfeeding on demand day and night. ■ Ask the mother to alert you if breastfeeding difficulty. ■ Assess breastfeeding in every baby before planning for discharge. ■ **DO NOT** discharge if baby is not yet feeding well.	■ If mother reports breastfeeding difficulty, assess breastfeeding and help the mother with positioning and attachment **J3**.
■ Teach the mother how to care for the baby. → Keep the baby warm **K9**. → Give cord care **K10**. → Ensure hygiene **K10**. **DO NOT** expose the baby in direct sun. **DO NOT** put the baby on any cold surface. **DO NOT** bath the baby before 6 hours.	■ If the mother is unable to take care of the baby, provide care or teach the companion **K9-K10**. ■ Wash hands before and after handling the baby.
■ Ask the mother and companion to watch the baby and alert you if → Feet cold. → Breathing difficulty: grunting, fast or slow breathing, chest in-drawing. → Any bleeding.	■ If feet are cold: → Teach the mother to put the baby skin-to-skin **K13**. → Reassess in 1 hour; if feet still cold, measure temperature and re-warm the baby **K9**. ■ If bleeding from cord, check if tie is loose and retie the cord. ■ If other bleeding, assess the baby immediately **J2-J7**. ■ If breathing difficulty or mother reports any other abnormality, examine the baby as on **J2-J7**.
■ Give prescribed treatments according to the schedule **K12**.	
■ Examine every baby before planning to discharge mother and baby **J2-J9**. **DO NOT** discharge before baby is 24 hours old.	

▼ **Next:** Additional care of a small baby (or twin)

ADDITIONAL CARE OF A SMALL BABY (OR TWIN)

Use this chart for additional care of a small baby: preterm, 1-2 months early or weighing 1500 g-<2500 g. Refer to hospital a very small baby: >2 months early, weighing <1500 g

CARE AND MONITORING

- Plan to keep the small baby longer before discharging.
- Allow visits to the mother and baby.

- Give special support for breastfeeding the small baby (or twins) K4:
  → Encourage the mother to breastfeed every 2-3 hours.
  → Assess breastfeeding daily: attachment, suckling, duration and frequency of feeds, and baby satisfaction with the feed J4 K6.
  → If alternative feeding method is used, assess the total daily amount of milk given.
  → Weigh daily and assess weight gain K7.

- Ensure additional warmth for the small baby K9:
  → Ensure the room is very warm (25°–28°C).
  → Teach the mother how to keep the small baby warm in skin-to-skin contact.
  → Provide extra blankets for mother and baby.
- Ensure hygiene K10.
  DO NOT bath the small baby. Wash as needed.

- Assess the small baby daily:
  → Measure temperature
  → Assess breathing (baby must be quiet, not crying): listen for grunting; count breaths per minute, repeat the count if >60 or <30; look for chest in-drawing
  → Look for jaundice (first 10 days of life): first 24 hours on the abdomen, then on palms and soles.

- Plan to discharge when:
  → Breastfeeding well
  → Gaining weight adequately on 3 consecutive days
  → Body temperature between 36.5° and 37.5°C on 3 consecutive days
  → Mother able and confident in caring for the baby
  → No maternal concerns.
- Assess the baby for discharge.

RESPOND TO ABNORMAL FINDINGS

- If the small baby is not suckling effectively and does not have other danger signs, consider alternative feeding methods K5-K6.
  → Teach the mother how to hand express breast milk directly into the baby's mouth K5
  → Teach the mother to express breast milk and cup feed the baby K5-K6
  → Determine appropriate amount for daily feeds by age K6.
- If feeding difficulty persists for 3 days, or weight loss greater than 10% of birth weight and no other problems, refer for breastfeeding counselling and management.

- If difficult to keep body temperature within the normal range (36.5°C to 37.5°C):
  → Keep the baby in skin-to-skin contact with the mother as much as possible
  → If body temperature below 36.5°C persists for 2 hours despite skin-to-skin contact with mother, assess the baby J2-J8.
- If breathing difficulty, assess the baby J2-J8.
- If jaundice, refer the baby for phototherapy.
- If any maternal concern, assess the baby and respond to the mother J2-J8.

- If the mother and baby are not able to stay, ensure daily (home) visits or send to hospital.

Additional care of a small baby (or twin) — J11

Assess replacement feeding

J12

ASSESS REPLACEMENT FEEDING

If mother chose replacement feeding assess the feeding in every baby as part of the examination.
Advise the mother on how to relieve engorgement K8 . **If mother is complaining of breast pain, also assess the mother's breasts** J9 .

ASK, CHECK RECORD

Ask the mother
- What are you feeding the baby?
- How are you feeding your baby?
- Has your baby fed in the previous hour?
- Is there any difficulty?
- How much milk is baby taking per feed?
- Is your baby satisfied with the feed?
- Have you fed your baby any other foods or drinks?
- Do you have any concerns?

If baby more than one day old:
- How many times has your baby fed in 24 hours?
- How much milk is baby taking per day?
- How do your breasts feel?

LOOK, LISTEN, FEEL

Observe a feed
- If the baby has not fed in the previous hour, ask the mother to feed the baby and observe feeding for about 5 minutes. Ask her to prepare the feed.

Look
- Is she holding the cup to the baby's lips?
- Is the baby alert, opens eyes and mouth?
- Is the baby sucking and swallowing the milk effectively, spilling little?

If mother has fed in the last hour, ask her to tell you when her baby is willing to feed again.

SIGNS	CLASSIFY	TREAT AND ADVISE
■ Not sucking (after 6 hours of age). ■ Stopped feeding.	**NOT ABLE TO FEED**	■ Refer baby urgently to hospital K14 .
■ Not yet fed (first 6 hours of life). ■ Not fed by cup. ■ Not sucking and swallowing effectively, spilling ■ Not feeding adequate amount per day. ■ Feeding less than 8 times per 24 hours. ■ Receiving other foods or drinks. ■ Several days old and inadequate weight gain.	**FEEDING DIFFICULTY**	■ Teach the mother replacement feeding G8 . ■ Teach the mother cup feeding K6 . ■ Advise to feed more frequently, on demand, day and night. ■ Advise the mother to stop feeding the baby other foods or drinks or by bottle. ■ Reassess at the next feed or follow-up visit in 2 days.
■ Sucking and swallowing adequate amount of milk, spilling little. ■ Feeding 8 times in 24 hours on demand day and night.	**FEEDING WELL**	■ Encourage the mother to continue feeding by cup on demand K6 .

BREASTFEEDING, CARE, PREVENTIVE MEASURES AND TREATMENT FOR THE NEWBORN

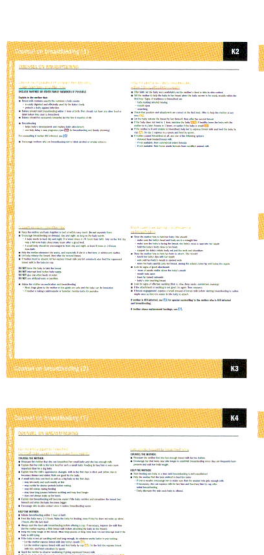

K2 COUNSEL ON BREASTFEEDING (1)
Counsel on importance of exclusive breast feeding
Help the mother to initiate breastfeeding

K3 COUNSEL ON BREASTFEEDING (2)
Support exclusive breastfeeding
Teach correct positioning and attachment for breastfeeding

K4 COUNSEL ON BREASTFEEDING (3)
Give special support to breastfeed the small baby (preterm and/or low birth weight)
Give special support to breastfeed twins

K5 ALTERNATIVE FEEDING METHODS (1)
Express breast milk
Hand express breast milk directly into the baby's mouth
Teach mother heat treating expressed breast milk

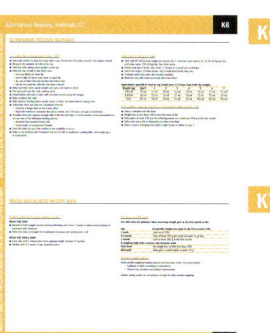

K6 ALTERNATIVE FEEDING METHODS (2)
Cup feeding expressed breast milk
Quantity to feed by cup
Signs that baby is receiving adequate amount of milk

K7 WEIGH AND ASSESS WEIGHT GAIN
Weigh baby in the first month of life
Assess weight gain
Scale maintenance

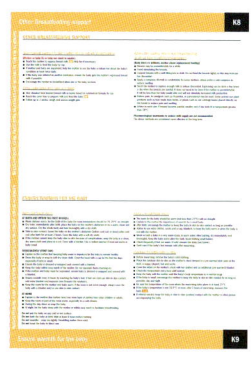

K8 OTHER BREASTFEEDING SUPPORT
Give special support to the mother who is not yet breastfeeding
Advise the mother who is not breastfeeding at all on how to relieve engorgement
If the baby does not have a mother

K9 ENSURE WARMTH FOR THE BABY
Keep the baby warm
Keep a small baby warm
Rewarm the baby skin-to-skin

K10 OTHER BABY CARE
Cord care
Sleeping
Hygiene

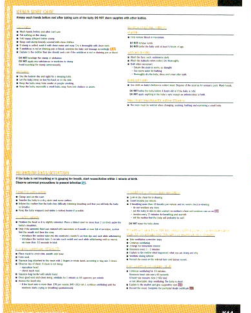

K11 NEWBORN RESUSCITATION
Keep the baby warm
Open the airway
If still not breathing, ventilate...
If breathing or crying, stop ventilating
If not breathing or gasping at all after 20 minutes of ventilation

K12 TREAT AND IMMUNIZE THE BABY (1)
Treat the baby
Give vitamin K
Give 2 IM antibiotics (first week of life)
Give IM benzathine penicillin to baby (single dose) if mother tested RPR positive
Give IM antibiotic for possible gonococcal eye infection (single dose)

K13 TREAT AND IMMUNIZE THE BABY (2)
Treat local infection
Provide eye care
Give isoniazid (INH) prophylaxis to newborn
Immunize the newborn

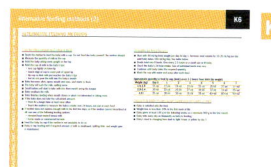

K14 ADVISE WHEN TO RETURN WITH THE BABY
Routine visits
Follow-up visits
Advise the mother to seek care for the baby
Refer baby urgently to hospital

- This section has details on breastfeeding, care of the baby, treatments, immunization, routine and follow-up visits and urgent referral to hospital.
- General principles are found in the section on good care `A1-A6`.
- If mother HIV-infected, see also `G7-G11`.

Counsel on breastfeeding (1) — K2

COUNSEL ON BREASTFEEDING

Counsel on importance of exclusive breastfeeding during pregnancy and after birth

INCLUDE PARTNER OR OTHER FAMILY MEMBERS IF POSSIBLE

Explain to the mother that:

- Breast milk contains exactly the nutrients a baby needs
  → is easily digested and efficiently used by the baby's body.
  → protects a baby against infection.
- Babies should start breastfeeding within 1 hour of birth. They should not have any other food or drink before they start to breastfeed.
- Babies should be exclusively breastfed for the first 6 months of life.
- Breastfeeding
  → helps baby's development and mother/baby attachment.
  → can help delay a new pregnancy (see **D27** for breastfeeding and family planning).

For counselling if mother HIV-infected, see **G7**.

- Encourage mothers who are breastfeeding not to drink alcohol or smoke tobacco.

Help the mother to initiate breastfeeding within 1 hour, when baby is ready

- After birth, let the baby rest comfortably on the mother's chest in skin-to-skin contact.
- Tell the mother to help the baby to her breast when the baby seems to be ready, usually within the first hour. Signs of readiness to breastfeed are:
  → baby looking around/moving
  → mouth open
  → searching.
- Check that position and attachment are correct at the first feed. Offer to help the mother at any time **K3**.
- Let the baby release the breast by her/himself; then offer the second breast.
- If the baby does not feed in 1 hour, examine the baby **J2–J9**. If healthy, leave the baby with the mother to try later. Assess in 3 hours, or earlier if the baby is small **J4**.
- If the mother is ill and unable to breastfeed, help her to express breast milk and feed the baby by cup **K6**. On day 1 express in a spoon and feed by spoon.
- If mother cannot breastfeed at all, use one of the following options:
  → donated heat-treated breast milk.
  → If not available, then commercial infant formula.
  → If not available, then home-made formula from modified animal milk.

Support exclusive breastfeeding

- Keep the mother and baby together in bed or within easy reach. **Do not** separate them.
- Encourage breastfeeding on demand, day and night, as long as the baby wants.
  → A baby needs to feed day and night, 8 or more times in 24 hours from birth. Only on the first day may a full-term baby sleep many hours after a good feed.
  → A small baby should be encouraged to feed, day and night, at least 8 times in 24 hours from birth.
- Help the mother whenever she wants, and especially if she is a first time or adolescent mother.
- Let baby release the breast, then offer the second breast.
- If mother must be absent, let her express breast milk and let somebody else feed the expressed breast milk to the baby by cup.

DO NOT force the baby to take the breast.
DO NOT interrupt feed before baby wants.
DO NOT give any other feeds or water.
DO NOT use artificial teats or pacifiers.

- Advise the mother on medication and breastfeeding
  → Most drugs given to the mother in this guide are safe and the baby can be breastfed.
  → If mother is taking cotrimoxazole or fansidar, monitor baby for jaundice.

Teach correct positioning and attachment for breastfeeding

- Show the mother how to hold her baby. She should:
  → make sure the baby's head and body are in a straight line
  → make sure the baby is facing the breast, the baby's nose is opposite her nipple
  → hold the baby's body close to her body
  → support the baby's whole body, not just the neck and shoulders
- Show the mother how to help her baby to attach. She should:
  → touch her baby's lips with her nipple
  → wait until her baby's mouth is opened wide
  → move her baby quickly onto her breast, aiming the infant's lower lip well below the nipple.
- Look for signs of good attachment:
  → more of areola visible above the baby's mouth
  → mouth wide open
  → lower lip turned outwards
  → baby's chin touching breast
- Look for signs of effective suckling (that is, slow, deep sucks, sometimes pausing).
- If the attachment or suckling is not good, try again. Then reassess.
- If breast engorgement, express a small amount of breast milk before starting breastfeeding to soften nipple area so that it is easier for the baby to attach.

If mother is HIV-infected, see G7 **for special counselling to the mother who is HIV-infected and breastfeeding.**

If mother chose replacement feedings, see G8.

Counsel on breastfeeding (2)

Counsel on breastfeeding (3)

K4

COUNSEL ON BREASTFEEDING

Give special support to breastfeed the small baby (preterm and/or low birth weight)

COUNSEL THE MOTHER:
- Reassure the mother that she can breastfeed her small baby and she has enough milk.
- Explain that her milk is the best food for such a small baby. Feeding for her/him is even more important than for a big baby.
- Explain how the milk's appearance changes: milk in the first days is thick and yellow, then it becomes thinner and whiter. Both are good for the baby.
- A small baby does not feed as well as a big baby in the first days:
  → may tire easily and suck weakly at first
  → may suckle for shorter periods before resting
  → may fall asleep during feeding
  → may have long pauses between suckling and may feed longer
  → does not always wake up for feeds.
- Explain that breastfeeding will become easier if the baby suckles and stimulates the breast her/himself and when the baby becomes bigger.
- Encourage skin-to-skin contact since it makes breastfeeding easier.

HELP THE MOTHER:
- Initiate breastfeeding within 1 hour of birth.
- Feed the baby every 2-3 hours. Wake the baby for feeding, even if she/he does not wake up alone, 2 hours after the last feed.
- Always start the feed with breastfeeding before offering a cup. If necessary, improve the milk flow (let the mother express a little breast milk before attaching the baby to the breast).
- Keep the baby longer at the breast. Allow long pauses or long, slow feed. Do not interrupt feed if the baby is still trying.
- If the baby is not yet suckling well and long enough, do whatever works better in your setting:
  → Let the mother express breast milk into baby's mouth **K5**.
  → Let the mother express breast milk and feed baby by cup **K6**. On the first day express breast milk into, and feed colostrum by spoon.
- Teach the mother to observe swallowing if giving expressed breast milk.
- Weigh the baby daily (if accurate and precise scales available), record and assess weight gain **K7**.

Give special support to breastfeed twins

COUNSEL THE MOTHER:
- Reassure the mother that she has enough breast milk for two babies.
- Encourage her that twins may take longer to establish breastfeeding since they are frequently born preterm and with low birth weight.

HELP THE MOTHER:
- Start feeding one baby at a time until breastfeeding is well established.
- Help the mother find the best method to feed the twins:
  → If one is weaker, encourage her to make sure that the weaker twin gets enough milk.
  → If necessary, she can express milk for her/him and feed her/him by cup after initial breastfeeding.
  → Daily alternate the side each baby is offered.

ALTERNATIVE FEEDING METHODS

Express breast milk

- The mother needs clean containers to collect and store the milk. A wide necked jug, jar, bowl or cup can be used.
- Once expressed, the milk should be stored with a well-fitting lid or cover.
- Teach the mother to express breast milk:
  - → To provide milk for the baby when she is away. To feed the baby if the baby is small and too weak to suckle
  - → To relieve engorgement and to help baby to attach
  - → To drain the breast when she has severe mastitis or abscesses.
- Teach the mother to express her milk by herself. **DO NOT** do it for her.
- Teach her how to:
  - → Wash her hands thoroughly.
  - → Sit or stand comfortably and hold a clean container underneath her breast.
  - → Put her first finger and thumb on either side of the areola, behind the nipple.
  - → Press slightly inwards towards the breast between her finger and thumb.
  - → Express one side until the milk flow slows. Then express the other side.
  - → Continue alternating sides for at least 20-30 minutes.
- Feed the baby by cup immediately. If not, store expressed milk in a cool, clean and safe place, at room temperature (8 hours) and in fridge (24 hours).
- If milk does not flow well:
  - → Apply warm compresses.
  - → Have someone massage her back and neck before expressing.
  - → Teach the mother breast and nipple massage.
  - → Feed the baby by cup immediately. If not, store expressed milk in a cool, clean and safe place.
- If necessary, repeat the procedure to express breast milk at least 8 times in 24 hours. Express as much as the baby would take or more, every 3 hours.
- When not breastfeeding at all, express just a little to relieve pain K5.
- If mother is very ill, help her to express or do it for her.

Hand express breast milk directly into the baby's mouth

- Teach the mother to express breast milk.
- Hold the baby in skin-to-skin contact, the mouth close to the nipple.
- Express the breast until some drops of breast milk appear on the nipple.
- Wait until the baby is alert and opens mouth and eyes, or stimulate the baby lightly to awaken her/him.
- Let the baby smell and lick the nipple, and attempt to suck.
- Let some breast milk fall into the baby's mouth.
- Wait until the baby swallows before expressing more drops of breast milk.
- After some time, when the baby has had enough, she/he will close her/his mouth and take no more breast milk.
- Ask the mother to repeat this process every 1-2 hours if the baby is very small (or every 2-3 hours if the baby is not very small).
- Be flexible at each feed, but make sure the intake is adequate by checking daily weight gain.

Teach mother heat treating expressed breast milk

Explain carefully and demonstrate how to heat treat expressed breast milk. Watch the mother practice the heat treating expressed breast milk. Check mother's understanding before she leaves.

- Express breast milk (50 to 150 ml) in a clean glass jar of 450 ml and close it with a lid.
- Label the jar with baby's name, the date and time.
- Place jar in a pot (around 1 litre) and pour boiling water in the pot – 450 ml or 2 cm below pot brim. If the jar is floating put weight on top of jar.
- Leave standing for ½hr. Remove milk, cool, feed the baby or store in fridge.

Alternative feeding methods (2)

K6

ALTERNATIVE FEEDING METHODS

Cup feeding expressed breast milk

- Teach the mother to feed the baby with a cup. Do not feed the baby yourself. The mother should:
- Measure the quantity of milk in the cup
- Hold the baby sitting semi-upright on her lap
- Hold the cup of milk to the baby's lips:
  → rest cup lightly on lower lip
  → touch edge of cup to outer part of upper lip
  → tip cup so that milk just reaches the baby's lips
  → but do not pour the milk into the baby's mouth.
- Baby becomes alert, opens mouth and eyes, and starts to feed.
- The baby will suck the milk, spilling some.
- Small babies will start to take milk into their mouth using the tongue.
- Baby swallows the milk.
- Baby finishes feeding when mouth closes or when not interested in taking more.
- If the baby does not take the calculated amount:
  → Feed for a longer time or feed more often
  → Teach the mother to measure the baby's intake over 24 hours, not just at each feed.
- If mother does not express enough milk in the first few days, or if the mother cannot breastfeed at all, use one of the following feeding options:
  → donated heat-treated breast milk
  → home-made or commercial formula.
- Feed the baby by cup if the mother is not available to do so.
- Baby is cup feeding well if required amount of milk is swallowed, spilling little, and weight gain is maintained.

Quantity to feed by cup

- Start with 80 ml/kg body weight per day for day 1. Increase total volume by 10-20 ml/kg per day, until baby takes 150 ml/kg/day. See table below.
- Divide total into 8 feeds. Give every 2-3 hours to a small size or ill baby.
- Check the baby's 24 hour intake. Size of individual feeds may vary.
- Continue until baby takes the required quantity.
- Wash the cup with water and soap after each feed.

Approximate quantity to feed by cup (in ml) every 2-3 hours from birth (by weight)

Weight (kg)	Day 0	1	2	3	4	5	6	7
1.5-1.9	15 ml	17 ml	19 ml	21 ml	23 ml	25 ml	27 ml	27+ml
2.0-2.4	20 ml	22 ml	25 ml	27 ml	30 ml	32 ml	35 ml	35+ml
2.5+	25 ml	28 ml	30 ml	35 ml	35 ml	40+ml	45+ml	50+ml

Signs that baby is receiving adequate amount of milk

- Baby is satisfied with the feed.
- Weight loss is less than 10% in the first week of life.
- Baby gains at least 160 g in the following weeks or a minimum 300 g in the first month.
- Baby wets every day as frequently as baby is feeding.
- Baby's stool is changing from dark to light brown or yellow by day 3.

WEIGH AND ASSESS WEIGHT GAIN

Weigh baby in the first month of life

WEIGH THE BABY
- Monthly if birth weight normal and breastfeeding well. Every 2 weeks if replacement feeding or treatment with isoniazid.
- When the baby is brought for examination because not feeding well, or ill.

WEIGH THE SMALL BABY
- Every day until 3 consecutive times gaining weight (at least 15 g/day).
- Weekly until 4-6 weeks of age (reached term).

Assess weight gain

Use this table for guidance when assessing weight gain in the first month of life

Age	Acceptable weight loss/gain in the first month of life
1 week	Loss up to 10%
2-4 weeks	Gain at least 160 g per week (at least 15 g/day)
1 month	Gain at least 300 g in the first month
If weighing daily with a precise and accurate scale	
First week	No weight loss or total less than 10%
Afterward	daily gain in small babies at least 20 g

Scale maintenance

Daily/weekly weighing requires precise and accurate scale (10 g increment):
→ Calibrate it daily according to instructions.
→ Check it for accuracy according to instructions.

Simple spring scales are not precise enough for daily/weekly weighing.

Other Breastfeeding support

K8

OTHER BREASTFEEDING SUPPORT

Give special support to the mother who is not yet breastfeeding

(Mother or baby ill, or baby too small to suckle)
- Teach the mother to express breast milk **K5**. Help her if necessary.
- Use the milk to feed the baby by cup.
- If mother and baby are separated, help the mother to see the baby or inform her about the baby's condition at least twice daily.
- If the baby was referred to another institution, ensure the baby gets the mother's expressed breast milk if possible.
- Encourage the mother to breastfeed when she or the baby recovers.

If the baby does not have a mother

- Give donated heat treated breast milk or home-based or commercial formula by cup.
- Teach the carer how to prepare milk and feed the baby **K6**.
- Follow up in 2 weeks; weigh and assess weight gain.

Advise the mother who is not breastfeeding at all on how to relieve engorgement

(Baby died or stillborn, mother chose replacement feeding)
- Breasts may be uncomfortable for a while.
- Avoid stimulating the breasts.
- Support breasts with a well-fitting bra or cloth. Do not bind the breasts tightly as this may increase her discomfort.
- Apply a compress. Warmth is comfortable for some mothers, others prefer a cold compress to reduce swelling.
- Teach the mother to express enough milk to relieve discomfort. Expressing can be done a few times a day when the breasts are overfull. It does not need to be done if the mother is uncomfortable. It will be less than her baby would take and will not stimulate increased milk production.
- Relieve pain. An analgesic such as ibuprofen, or paracetamol may be used. Some women use plant products such as teas made from herbs, or plants such as raw cabbage leaves placed directly on the breast to reduce pain and swelling.
- Advise to seek care if breasts become painful, swollen, red, if she feels ill or temperature greater than 38°C.

Pharmacological treatments to reduce milk supply are not recommended.
The above methods are considered more effective in the long term.

ENSURE WARMTH FOR THE BABY

Keep the baby warm

AT BIRTH AND WITHIN THE FIRST HOUR(S)
- Warm delivery room: for the birth of the baby the room temperature should be 25-28°C, no draught.
- Dry baby: immediately after birth, place the baby on the mother's abdomen or on a warm, clean and dry surface. Dry the whole body and hair thoroughly, with a dry cloth.
- Skin-to-skin contact: Leave the baby on the mother's abdomen (before cord cut) or chest (after cord cut) after birth for at least 2 hours. Cover the baby with a soft dry cloth.
- If the mother cannot keep the baby skin-to-skin because of complications, wrap the baby in a clean, dry, warm cloth and place in a cot. Cover with a blanket. Use a radiant warmer if room not warm or baby small.

SUBSEQUENTLY (FIRST DAY)
- Explain to the mother that keeping baby warm is important for the baby to remain healthy.
- Dress the baby or wrap in soft dry clean cloth. Cover the head with a cap for the first few days, especially if baby is small.
- Ensure the baby is dressed or wrapped and covered with a blanket.
- Keep the baby within easy reach of the mother. Do not separate them (rooming-in).
- If the mother and baby must be separated, ensure baby is dressed or wrapped and covered with a blanket.
- Assess warmth every 4 hours by touching the baby's feet: if feet are cold use skin-to-skin contact, add extra blanket and reassess (see Rewarm the newborn).
- Keep the room for the mother and baby warm. If the room is not warm enough, always cover the baby with a blanket and/or use skin-to-skin contact.

AT HOME
- Explain to the mother that babies need one more layer of clothes than other children or adults.
- Keep the room or part of the room warm, especially in a cold climate.
- During the day, dress or wrap the baby.
- At night, let the baby sleep with the mother or within easy reach to facilitate breastfeeding.

Do not put the baby on any cold or wet surface.
Do not bath the baby at birth. Wait at least 6 hours before bathing.
Do not swaddle – wrap too tightly. Swaddling makes them cold.
Do not leave the baby in direct sun.

Keep a small baby warm

- The room for the baby should be warm (not less than 25°C) with no draught.
- Explain to the mother the importance of warmth for a small baby.
- After birth, encourage the mother to keep the baby in skin-to-skin contact as long as possible.
- Advise to use extra clothes, socks and a cap, blankets, to keep the baby warm or when the baby is not with the mother.
- Wash or bath a baby in a very warm room, in warm water. After bathing, dry immediately and thoroughly. Keep the baby warm after the bath. Avoid bathing small babies.
- Check frequently if feet are warm. If cold, rewarm the baby (see below).
- Seek care if the baby's feet remain cold after rewarming.

Rewarm the baby skin-to-skin

- Before rewarming, remove the baby's cold clothing.
- Place the newborn skin-to-skin on the mother's chest dressed in a pre-warmed shirt open at the front, a nappy (diaper), hat and socks.
- Cover the infant on the mother's chest with her clothes and an additional (pre-warmed) blanket.
- Check the temperature every hour until normal.
- Keep the baby with the mother until the baby's body temperature is in normal range.
- If the baby is small, encourage the mother to keep the baby in skin-to-skin contact for as long as possible, day and night.
- Be sure the temperature of the room where the rewarming takes place is at least 25°C.
- If the baby's temperature is not 36.5°C or more after 2 hours of rewarming, reassess the baby J2-J7.
- If referral needed, keep the baby in skin-to-skin position/contact with the mother or other person accompanying the baby.

Other baby care

K10

OTHER BABY CARE

Always wash hands before and after taking care of the baby. DO NOT share supplies with other babies.

Cord care

- Wash hands before and after cord care.
- Put nothing on the stump.
- Fold nappy (diaper) below stump.
- Keep cord stump loosely covered with clean clothes.
- If stump is soiled, wash it with clean water and soap. Dry it thoroughly with clean cloth.
- If umbilicus is red or draining pus or blood, examine the baby and manage accordingly `J2-J7`.
- Explain to the mother that she should seek care if the umbilicus is red or draining pus or blood.

   DO NOT bandage the stump or abdomen.
   DO NOT apply any substances or medicine to stump.
   Avoid touching the stump unnecessarily.

Sleeping

- Use the bednet day and night for a sleeping baby.
- Let the baby sleep on her/his back or on the side.
- Keep the baby away from smoke or people smoking.
- Keep the baby, especially a small baby, away from sick children or adults.

Hygiene (washing, bathing)

AT BIRTH:

- Only remove blood or meconium.

   DO NOT remove vernix.
   DO NOT bathe the baby until at least 6 hours of age.

LATER AND AT HOME:

- Wash the face, neck, underarms daily.
- Wash the buttocks when soiled. Dry thoroughly.
- Bath when necessary:
   → Ensure the room is warm, no draught
   → Use warm water for bathing
   → Thoroughly dry the baby, dress and cover after bath.

OTHER BABY CARE:

- Use cloth on baby's bottom to collect stool. Dispose of the stool as for woman's pads. Wash hands.

   DO NOT bathe the baby before 6 hours old or if the baby is cold.
   DO NOT apply anything in the baby's eyes except an antimicrobial at birth.

SMALL BABIES REQUIRE MORE CAREFUL ATTENTION:

- The room must be warmer when changing, washing, bathing and examining a small baby.

NEWBORN RESUSCITATION

If the baby is not breathing or is gasping for breath, start resuscitation within 1 minute of birth.
Observe universal precautions to prevent infection A4.

Keep the baby warm

- Clamp and cut the cord.
- Transfer the baby to a dry, clean and warm surface.
- Inform the mother that the baby has difficulty initiating breathing and that you will help the baby to breathe.
- Keep the baby wrapped and under a radiant heater if possible.

Open the airway

- Position the head so it is slightly extended. Place a folded towel no more than 2 cm thick under the baby's shoulders.
- In neonates born through clear amniotic fluid who do not start breathing after thorough drying and rubbing the back 2-3 times, suctioning of the mouth and nose should not be done routinely before initiating positive pressure ventilation.
- Suctioning should be done only if the mouth or nose is full of secretions.
- full of secretions.
  → Introduce the suction tube into the newborn's mouth 5 cm from lips and suck while withdrawing.
  → Introduce the suction tube 3 cm into each nostril and suck while withdrawing until no mucus, no more than 10 seconds in total.

If still no breathing, VENTILATE:

- Place mask to cover chin, mouth, and nose.
- Form seal.
- Squeeze bag attached to the mask with 2 fingers or whole hand, according to bag size, 5 times.
- Observe rise of chest. If chest is not rising:
  → reposition head
  → check mask seal.
- Squeeze bag harder with whole hand.
- Once good seal and chest rising, ventilate for 1 minute at 40 squeezes per minute.
- Assess the heart rate
  → if the heart rate is more than 100 per minute (HR>100/min.), continue ventilating until the newborn starts crying or breathing spontaneously.

If breathing or crying, stop ventilating

- Look at the chest for in-drawing.
- Count breaths per minute.
- If breathing more than 30 breaths per minute and no severe chest in-drawing:
  → do not ventilate any more
  → put the baby in skin-to-skin contact on mother's chest and continue care as on D19
  → monitor every 15 minutes for breathing and warmth
  → tell the mother that the baby will probably be well.

- **DO NOT** leave the baby alone

If heart rate less than 100 per minute (HR<100/min.) or breathing less than 30 per minute (RR<30/min.) or severe chest in-drawing:

- Take ventilation corrective steps
- Continue ventilating.
- Arrange for immediate referral.
- Reassess every 1 - 2 minutes
- Explain to the mother what happened, what you are doing and why.
- Ventilate during referral.
- Record the event on the referral form and labour record.

If no breathing or gasping at all

- Continue ventilating for 10 minutes.
  Reassess heart rate every 60 seconds.
  If heart rate remains slow (<60/min) or not detectable, stop ventilating. The baby is dead.
- Explain to the mother and give supportive care D24.
- Record the event. Complete the perinatal death certificate N7.

Treat and immunize the baby (1)

K12

TREAT THE BABY

Treat the baby

- Determine appropriate drugs and dosage for the baby's weight.
- Give 1 mg of vitamin K IM to all newborns, one hour after birth.
- Tell the mother the reasons for giving the drug to the baby.
- Give intramuscular antibiotics in thigh. Use a new syringe and needle for each antibiotic.

Give 2 IM antibiotics (first week of life)

- Give first dose of both ampicillin and gentamicin IM in thigh before referral for possible serious illness, severe umbilical infection or severe skin infection.
- Give both ampicillin and gentamicin IM for 5 days in asymptomatic babies classified at risk of infection.
- Give intramuscular antibiotics in thigh. Use a new syringe and needle for each antibiotic.

Weight	**Ampicillin IM** Dose: 50 mg perkg every 12 hours Add 2.5 ml sterile water to 500 mg vial = 200 mg/ml	**Gentamicin IM** Dose: 5 mg perkg every 24 hours if term; 4 mg perkg every 24 hours if preterm 20 mg per 2 ml vial = 10 mg/ml
1.0 – 1.4 kg	0.35 ml	0.5 ml
1.5 – 1.9 kg	0.5 ml	0.7 ml
2.0 – 2.4 kg	0.6 ml	0.9 ml
2.5 – 2.9 kg	0.75 ml	1.35 ml
3.0 – 3.4 kg	0.85 ml	1.6 ml
3.5 – 3.9 kg	1 ml	1.85 ml
4.0 – 4.4 kg	1.1 ml	2.1 ml

Give IM benzathine penicillin to baby (single dose) if mother tested RPR-positive

Weight	**Benzathine penicillin IM** Dose: 50 000 units/kg once Add 5 ml sterile water to vial containing 1.2 million units = 1.2 million units/(6 ml total volume) = 200 000 units/ml
1.0 - 1.4 kg	0.35 ml
1.5 - 1.9 kg	0.5 ml
2.0 - 2.4 kg	0.6 ml
2.5 - 2.9 kg	0.75 ml
3.0 - 3.4 kg	0.85 ml
3.5 - 3.9 kg	1.0 ml
4.0 - 4.4 kg	1.1 ml

Give IM antibiotic for possible gonococcal eye infection (single dose)

Weight	**Ceftriaxone (1st choice)** Dose: 50 mg perkg once 250 mg per 5 ml vial=mg/ml	**Kanamycin (2nd choice)** Dose: 25 mg perkg once, max 75 mg 75 mg per 2 ml vial = 37.5 mg/ml
1.0 - 1.4 kg	1 ml	0.7 ml
1.5 - 1.9 kg	1.5 ml	1 ml
2.0 - 2.4 kg	2 ml	1.3 ml
2.5 - 2.9 kg	2.5 ml	1.7 ml
3.0 - 3.4 kg	3 ml	2 ml
3.5 - 3.9 kg	3.5 ml	2 ml
4.0 - 4.4 kg	4 ml	2 ml

Teach the mother to give treatment to the baby at home

- Explain carefully how to give the treatment. Label and package each drug separately.
- Check mother's understanding before she leaves the clinic.
- Demonstrate how to measure a dose.
- Watch the mother practice measuring a dose by herself.
- Watch the mother give the first dose to the baby.

Treat local infection

TEACH MOTHER TO TREAT LOCAL INFECTION

- Explain and show how the treatment is given.
- Watch her as she carries out the first treatment.
- Ask her to let you know if the local infection gets worse and to return to the clinic if possible.
- Treat for 5 days.

TREAT SKIN PUSTULES OR UMBILICAL INFECTION

- **Do the following 3 times daily:**
- Wash hands with clean water and soap.
- Gently wash off pus and crusts with boiled and cooled water and soap.
- Dry the area with clean cloth.
- Paint with gentian violet.
- Wash hands.

TREAT EYE INFECTION

Do the following 6-8 times daily:
- Wash hands with clean water and soap.
- Wet clean cloth with boiled and cooled water.
- Use the wet cloth to gently wash off pus from the baby's eyes.
- Apply 1% tetracycline eye ointment in each eye 3 times daily.
- Wash hands.

REASSESS IN 2 DAYS:

- Assess the skin, umbilicus or eyes.
- If pus or redness remains or is worse, refer to hospital.
- If pus and redness have improved, tell the mother to continue treating local infection at home.

Give isoniazid (INH) prophylaxis to newborn

If the mother is diagnosed as having tuberculosis and started treatment less than 2 months before delivery:
- Give 5 mg/kg isoniazid (INH) orally once a day for 6 months (1 tablet = 200 mg).
- Delay BCG vaccination until INH treatment completed, or repeat BCG.
- Reassure the mother that it is safe to breastfeed the baby.
- Follow up the baby every 2 weeks, or according to national guidelines, to assess weight gain.

Immunize the newborn

- Give BCG, OPV-0, Hepatitis B vaccine birth dose, within 24 hours after birth, preferably before discharge.
- If un-immunized newborn first seen 1-4 weeks of age, give BCG only.
- Record on immunization card and child record.
- Advise when to return for next immunization.

Age	Vaccine
Birth <1 week	BCG OPV-0 HB1
6 weeks	DPT OPV-1 HB-2

Give ARV drugs to the HIV-exposed newborn

- Give the first dose of ARV drugs to newborn 6–12 hours after birth G9, G12.
- Give Nevirapine 2 mg/kg once only.
- Give Zidovudine 4 mg/kg every 12 hours.
- If the newborn spills or vomits within 30 minutes repeat the dose.

Teach mother to give oral ARV drugs at home

- Explain and show how the drug is given.
- Wash hands.
- Demonstrate how to use the syringe and how to measure the dose.
- Ask the mother to begin breastfeeding or feed the baby by cup.
- Give drug by the syringe into the baby's mouth before the end of the feed.
- Complete the feed.
- Watch the mother as she carries out the next treatment.
- Explain to the mother that she should watch her baby after giving a dose of ARV drug. If baby vomits or spills within 30 minutes, she should repeat the dose.
- Tell her to give the ARV drugs every day at the same time for 6 weeks.
- Prescribe or give her enough ARV(s) until the next visit.

Treat and immunize the baby (2)

K13

Advise when to return with the baby K14

ADVISE WHEN TO RETURN WITH THE BABY

For maternal visits see schedule on D28.

Routine postnatal contacts

	Return
Postnatal visit	First visit (at home) at 3 days
	Second visit at 7-14 days
	At age 6 weeks
Immunization visit	At age 6 weeks
(If BCG, OPV-0 and HB-1 given in the first week of life)	

Follow-up visits

If the problem was:	Return in
Feeding difficulty	2 days
Red umbilicus	2 days
Skin infection	2 days
Eye infection	2 days
Thrush	2 days
Mother has either:	
→ breast engorgement or	2 days
→ mastitis.	2 days
Low birth weight, and either	
→ first week of life or	2 days
→ not adequately gaining weight	2 days
Low birth weight, and either	
→ older than 1 week or	7 days
→ gaining weight adequately	7 days
Orphan baby	14 days
INH prophylaxis	14 days
Treated for possible congenital syphilis	14 days
Mother HIV-infected	14 days

Advise the mother to seek care for the baby

Use the counselling sheet to advise the mother when to seek care, or when to return, if the baby has any of these danger signs:

RETURN OR GO TO THE HOSPITAL IMMEDIATELY IF THE BABY HAS

- difficulty breathing.
- convulsions.
- fever or feels cold.
- bleeding.
- diarrhoea.
- very small, just born.
- not feeding at all.

GO TO HEALTH CENTRE AS QUICKLY AS POSSIBLE IF THE BABY HAS

- difficulty feeding.
- pus from eyes.
- skin pustules.
- yellow skin.
- a cord stump which is red or draining pus.
- feeds <5 times in 24 hours.

Refer baby urgently to hospital

- After emergency treatment, explain the need for referral to the mother/father.
- Organize safe transportation.
- Always send the mother with the baby, if possible.
- Send referral note with the baby.
- Inform the referral centre if possible by radio or telephone.

DURING TRANSPORTATION

- Keep the baby warm by skin-to-skin contact with mother or someone else.
- Cover the baby with a blanket and cover her/his head with a cap.
- Protect the baby from direct sunshine.
- Encourage breastfeeding during the journey.
- If the baby does not breastfeed and journey is more than 3 hours, consider giving expressed breast milk by cup K6

EQUIPMENT, SUPPLIES, DRUGS AND LABORATORY TESTS

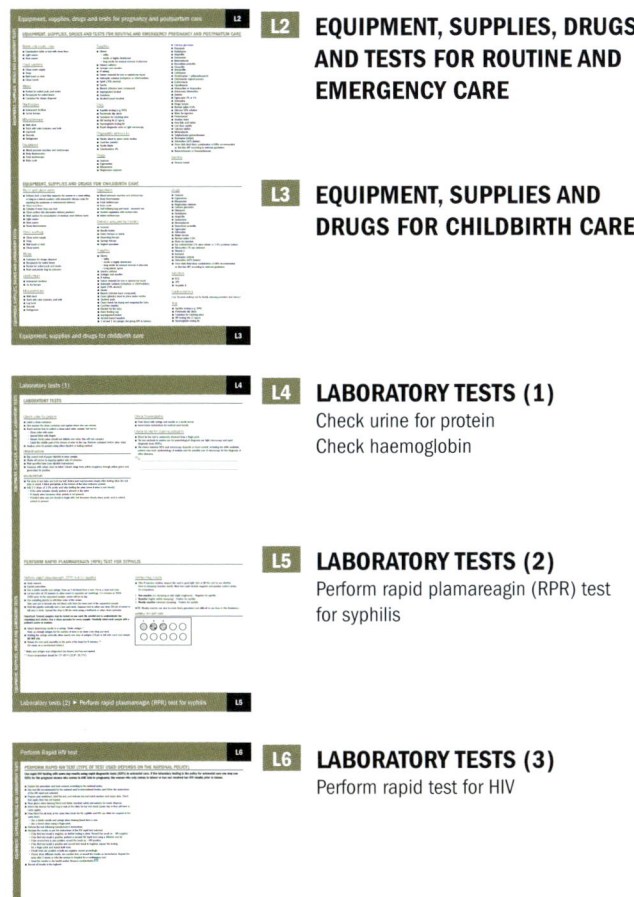

L2   **EQUIPMENT, SUPPLIES, DRUGS AND TESTS FOR ROUTINE AND EMERGENCY CARE**

L3   **EQUIPMENT, SUPPLIES AND DRUGS FOR CHILDBIRTH CARE**

L4   **LABORATORY TESTS (1)**
Check urine for protein
Check haemoglobin

L5   **LABORATORY TESTS (2)**
Perform rapid plamareagin (RPR) test for syphilis

L6   **LABORATORY TESTS (3)**
Perform rapid test for HIV

Equipment, supplies, drugs and laboratory tests

L1

Equipment, supplies, drugs and tests for pregnancy and postpartum care

EQUIPMENT, SUPPLIES, DRUGS AND TESTS FOR ROUTINE AND EMERGENCY PREGNANCY AND POSTPARTUM CARE

Warm and clean room

- Examination table or bed with clean linen
- Light source
- Heat source

Hand washing

- Clean water supply
- Soap
- Nail brush or stick
- Clean towels

Waste

- Bucket for soiled pads and swabs
- Receptacle for soiled linens
- Container for sharps disposal

Sterilization

- Instrument sterilizer
- Jar for forceps

Miscellaneous

- Wall clock
- Torch with extra batteries and bulb
- Log book
- Records
- Refrigerator

Equipment

- Blood pressure machine and stethoscope
- Body thermometer
- Fetal stethoscope
- Baby scale

Supplies

- Gloves:
  - → utility
  - → sterile or highly disinfected
  - → long sterile for manual removal of placenta
- Urinary catheter
- Syringes and needles
- IV tubing
- Suture material for tear or episiotomy repair
- Spirit (70% alcohol)
- Swabs
- Bleach (chlorine base compound)
- Impregnated bednet
- Condoms
- Alcohol-based handrub

Tests

- Syphilis testing (e.g. RPR)
- Proteinuria dip sticks
- Container for catching urine
- HIV testing kit (2 types)
- Haemoglobin testing kit
- Rapid diagnostic tests or Light microscopy

Disposable delivery kit

- Plastic sheet to place under mother
- Cord ties (sterile)
- Sterile blade
- 7.1% chlorhexidine digluconate (delivering 4% chlorhexidine) (gel or liquid) for umbilical cord care.

Drugs

- Oxytocin
- Ergometrine
- Misoprostol
- Magnesium sulphate
- Calcium gluconate
- Diazepam
- Hydralazine
- Ampicillin
- Gentamicin
- Metronidazole
- Benzathine penicillin
- Cloxacillin
- Amoxycillin
- Ceftriaxone
- Trimethoprim + sulfamethoxazole
- Clotrimazole vaginal pessary
- Erythromycin
- Ciprofloxacin
- Tetracycline or doxycycline
- Artesunate/Artemether
- Quinine
- Lignocaine 2% or 1%
- Adrenaline
- Ringer lactate
- Normal saline 0.9%
- Glucose 50% solution
- Water for injection
- Paracetamol
- Gentian violet
- Iron/folic acid tablet
- Low-dose aspirin
- Calcium tablets
- Mebendazole
- Sulphadoxine-pyrimethamine
- Nevirapine (infant)
- Zidovudine (AZT) (infant)
- Once-daily fixed-dose combination of ARVs recommended as first-line ART according to national guidelines
- Betamethasone or Dexamethasone

Vaccine

- Tetanus toxoid

EQUIPMENT, SUPPLIES AND DRUGS FOR CHILDBIRTH CARE

Warm and clean room

- Delivery bed: a bed that supports the woman in a semi-sitting or lying in a lateral position, with removable stirrups (only for repairing the perineum or instrumental delivery)
- Clean bed linen
- Curtains if more than one bed
- Clean surface (for alternative delivery position)
- Work surface for resuscitation of newborn near delivery beds
- Light source
- Heat source
- Room thermometer

Hand washing

- Clean water supply
- Soap
- Nail brush or stick
- Clean towels

Waste

- Container for sharps disposal
- Receptacle for soiled linens
- Bucket for soiled pads and swabs
- Bowl and plastic bag for placenta

Sterilization

- Instrument sterilizer
- Jar for forceps

Miscellaneous

- Wall clock
- Torch with extra batteries and bulb
- Log book
- Records
- Refrigerator

Equipment

- Blood pressure machine and stethoscope
- Body thermometer
- Fetal stethoscope
- Baby scale
- Self inflating bag and mask - neonatal size
- Suction apparatus with suction tube
- Infant stethoscope

Delivery instruments (sterile)

- Scissors
- Needle holder
- Artery forceps or clamp
- Dissecting forceps
- Sponge forceps
- Vaginal speculum

Supplies

- Gloves:
  → utility
  → sterile or highly disinfected
  → long sterile for manual removal of placenta
  → Long plastic apron
- Urinary catheter
- Syringes and needles
- IV tubing
- Suture material for tear or episiotomy repair
- Antiseptic solution (iodophors or chlorhexidine)
- Spirit (70% alcohol)
- Swabs
- Bleach (chlorine-base compound)
- Clean (plastic) sheet to place under mother
- Sanitary pads
- Clean towels for drying and wrapping the baby
- Cord ties (sterile)
- Blanket for the baby
- Baby feeding cup
- Impregnated bednet
- Alcohol-based handrub
- 2 ml and 1 ml syringes (for giving ARV to babies)

Drugs

- Oxytocin
- Ergometrine
- Misoprostol
- Magnesium sulphate
- Calcium gluconate
- Diazepam
- Hydralazine
- Ampicillin
- Gentamicin
- Benzathine penicillin
- Lignocaine
- Adrenaline
- Ringer lactate
- Normal saline 0.9%
- Water for injection
- Eye antimicrobial (1% silver nitrate or 2.5% povidone iodine)
- Tetracycline 1% eye ointment
- Vitamin K
- Izoniazid
- Nevirapine (infant)
- Zidovudine (AZT) (infant)
- Once-daily fixed-dose combination of ARVs recommended as first-line ART according to national guidelines

Vaccines

- BCG
- OPV
- Hepatitis B

Contraceptives

(see Decision-making tool for family planning providers and clients)

Test

- Syphilis testing (e.g. RPR)
- Proteinuria dip sticks
- Container for catching urine
- HIV testing kits (2 types)
- Haemoglobin testing kit

Laboratory tests (1) L4

LABORATORY TESTS

Check urine for protein

- Label a clean container.
- Give woman the clean container and explain where she can urinate.
- Teach woman how to collect a clean-catch urine sample. Ask her to:
  → Clean vulva with water
  → Spread labia with fingers
  → Urinate freely (urine should not dribble over vulva; this will ruin sample)
  → Catch the middle part of the stream of urine in the cup. Remove container before urine stops.
- Analyse urine for protein using either dipstick or boiling method.

DIPSTICK METHOD

- Dip coated end of paper dipstick in urine sample.
- Shake off excess by tapping against side of container.
- Wait specified time (see dipstick instructions).
- Compare with colour chart on label. Colours range from yellow (negative) through yellow-green and green-blue for positive.

BOILING METHOD

- Put urine in test tube and boil top half. Boiled part may become cloudy. After boiling allow the test tube to stand. A thick precipitate at the bottom of the tube indicates protein.
- Add 2-3 drops of 2-3% acetic acid after boiling the urine (even if urine is not cloudy)
  → If the urine remains cloudy, protein is present in the urine.
  → If cloudy urine becomes clear, protein is not present.
  → If boiled urine was not cloudy to begin with, but becomes cloudy when acetic acid is added, protein is present.

Check haemoglobin

- Draw blood with syringe and needle or a sterile lancet.
- Insert below instructions for method used locally.

Check blood for malaria parasites

- Blood for the test is commonly obtained from a finger-prick.
- The two methods in routine use for parasitological diagnosis are light microscopy and rapid diagnostic tests (RDTs).
- The choice between RDTs and microscopy depends on local context, including the skills available, patient case-load, epidemiology of malaria and the possible use of microscopy for the diagnosis of other diseases.

PERFORM RAPID PLASMAREAGIN (RPR) TEST FOR SYPHILIS

Perform rapid plasmareagin (RPR) test for syphilis

- Seek consent.
- Explain procedure.
- Use a sterile needle and syringe. Draw up 5 ml blood from a vein. Put in a clear test tube.
- Let test tube sit 20 minutes to allow serum to separate (or centrifuge 3-5 minutes at 2000–3000-rpm). In the separated sample, serum will be on top.
- Use sampling pipette to withdraw some of the serum.
  Take care not to include any red blood cells from the lower part of the separated sample.
- Hold the pipette vertically over a test card circle. Squeeze teat to allow one drop (50-µl) of serum to fall onto a circle. Spread the drop to fill the circle using a toothpick or other clean spreader.

Important: Several samples may be tested on one card. Be careful not to contaminate the remaining test circles. Use a clean spreader for every sample. Carefully label each sample with a patient's name or number.

- Attach dispensing needle to a syringe. Shake antigen.*
  Draw up enough antigen for the number of tests to be done (one drop per test).
- Holding the syringe vertically, allow exactly one drop of antigen (20-µl) to fall onto each test sample. **DO NOT stir.**
- Rotate the test card smoothly on the palm of the hand for 8 minutes.**
  (Or rotate on a mechanical rotator.)

* Make sure antigen was refrigerated (not frozen) and has not expired.
** Room temperature should be 73°-85°F (22.8°–29.3°C).

Interpreting results

- After 8 minutes rotation, inspect the card in good light. Turn or lift the card to see whether there is clumping (reactive result). Most test cards include negative and positive control circles for comparison.

1. **Non-reactive** (no clumping or only slight roughness) – Negative for syphilis
2. **Reactive** (highly visible clumping) - Positive for syphilis
3. **Weakly reactive** (minimal clumping) - Positive for syphilis

NOTE: Weakly reactive can also be more finely granulated and difficult to see than in this illsutration.

EXAMPLE OF A TEST CARD

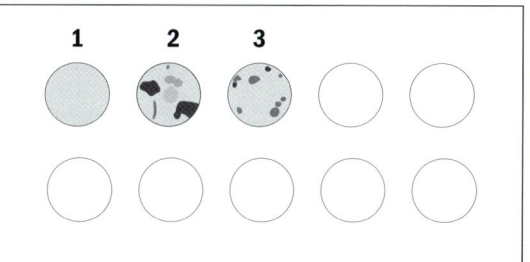

Perform Rapid HIV test

L6

PERFORM RAPID HIV TEST (TYPE OF TEST USED DEPENDS ON THE NATIONAL POLICY)

Use rapid HIV testing with same-day results using rapid diagnostic tests (RDTs) in antenatal care. If the laboratory testing is the policy for antenatal care you may use RDTs for the pregnant woman who comes to ANC late in pregnancy, the woman who only comes in labour or has not received her HIV results prior to labour.

- Explain the procedure and seek consent according to the national policy.
- Use test kits recommended by the national and/or international bodies and follow the instructions of the HIV rapid test selected.
- Prepare your worksheet, label the test, and indicate the test batch number and expiry date. Check that expiry time has not lapsed.
- Wear gloves when drawing blood and follow standard safety precautions for waste disposal.
- Inform the woman for how long to wait at the clinic for her test result (same day or they will have to come again).
- Draw blood for all tests at the same time (tests for Hb, syphilis and HIV can often be coupled at the same time).
  → Use a sterile needle and syringe when drawing blood from a vein.
  → Use a lancet when doing a finger prick.
- Perform the test following manufacturer's instructions.
- Interpret the results as per the instructions of the HIV rapid test selected.
  → If the first test result is negative, no further testing is done. Record the result as – HIV-negative.
  → If the first test result is positive, perform a second HIV rapid test using a different test kit.
  → If the second test is also positive, record the result as – HIV-positive.
  → If the first test result is positive and second test result is negative, repeat the testing. Do a finger prick and repeat both tests.
  → If both tests are positive or both are negative, record accordingly.
  → If tests show different results, use another test, or record the results as inconclusive. Repeat the tests after 2 weeks or refer the woman to hospital for a confirmatory test.
  → Send the results to the health worker. Respect confidentiality **A2**.
- Record all results in the logbook.

EQUIPMENT, SUPPLIES, DRUGS AND LABORATORY TESTS

INFORMATION AND COUNSELLING SHEETS

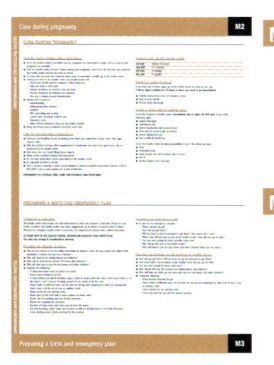

M2 CARE DURING PREGNANCY
Visit the health worker during pregnancy
Care for yourself during pregnancy
Routine visits to the health centre
Know the signs of labour
When to seek care on danger signs

M3 PREPARING A BIRTH AND EMERGENCY PLAN
Preparing a birth plan
Planning for delivery at home
Preparing an emergency plan
Planning for delivery at the hospital or health centre

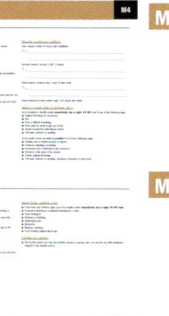

M4 CARE FOR THE MOTHER AFTER BIRTH
Care of the mother
Family planning
Routine visits to the health centre
When to seek care for danger signs

M5 CARE AFTER AN ABORTION
Self-care
Family planning
Know these DANGER signs
Additional support

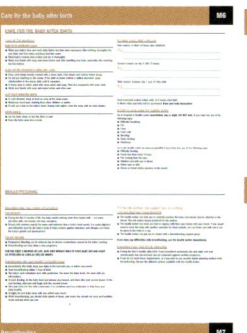

M6 CARE FOR THE BABY AFTER BIRTH
Care of the newborn
Routine visits to the health centre
When to seek care for danger signs

M7 BREASTFEEDING
Breastfeeding has many advantages for the baby and the mother
Suggestions for successful breastfeeding
Health worker support
Breastfeeding and family planning

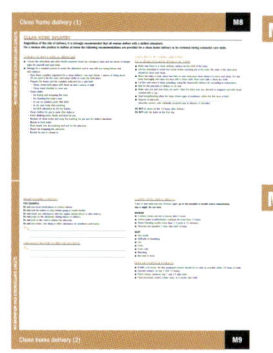

M8 CLEAN HOME DELIVERY (1)
Delivery at home with an attendant
Instructions to mother and family for a clean and safer delivery at home

M9 CLEAN HOME DELIVERY (2)
Avoid harmful practices
Encourage helpful traditional practices
Danger signs during delivery
Routine visits to the health centre

- These individual sheets have key information for the mother, her partner and family on care during pregnancy, preparing a birth and emergency plan, clean home delivery, care for the mother and baby after delivery, breastfeeding and care after an abortion.

- Individual sheets are used so that the woman can be given the relevant sheet at the appropriate stage of pregnancy and childbirth.

Information and counselling sheets

M1

Care during pregnancy

M2

CARE DURING PREGNANCY

Visit the health worker during pregnancy

- Go to the health centre if you think you are pregnant. It is important to begin care as early in your pregnancy as possible.
- Visit the health centre at least 4 times during your pregnancy, even if you do not have any problems. The health worker will tell you when to return.
- If at any time you have any concerns about your or your baby's health, go to the health centre.
- During your visits to the health centre, the health worker will:
  - → Check your health and the progress of the pregnancy
  - → Help you make a birth plan
  - → Answer questions or concerns you may have
  - → Provide treatment for malaria and anaemia
  - → Give you a tetanus toxoid immunization
- Advise and counsel on:
  - → breastfeeding
  - → birthspacing after delivery
  - → nutrition
  - → HIV counselling and testing
  - → correct and consistent condom use
  - → laboratory tests
  - → other matters related to your and your baby's health.
- Bring your home-based maternal record to every visit.

Care for yourself during pregnancy

- Eat more and healthier foods, including more fruits and vegetables, beans, meat, fish, eggs, cheese, milk.
- Take iron tablets and any other supplements or medicines you have been given every day as explained by the health worker.
- Rest when you can. Avoid lifting heavy objects.
- Sleep under a bednet treated with insecticide.
- Do not take medication unless prescribed at the health centre.
- Do not drink alcohol or smoke.
- Use a condom correctly in every sexual relation to prevent sexually transmitted infection (STI) or HIV/AIDS if you or your partner are at risk of infection.

PREGNANCY IS A SPECIAL TIME. CARE FOR YOURSELF AND YOUR BABY.

Routine visits to the health centre

1st visit	Before 4 months
2nd visit	6-7 months
3rd visit	8 months
4th visit	9 months

Know the signs of labour

If you have any of these signs, go to the health centre as soon as you can.
If these signs continue for 12 hours or more, you need to go immediately.

- Painful contractions every 20 minutes or less.
- Bag of water breaks.
- Bloody sticky discharge.

When to seek care on danger signs

Go to the hospital or health centre **immediately, day or night, DO NOT wait,** if any of the following signs:
- vaginal bleeding
- convulsions/fits
- severe headaches with blurred vision
- fever and too weak to get out of bed
- severe abdominal pain
- fast or difficult breathing.

Go to the health centre **as soon as possible** if any of the following signs:
- fever
- abdominal pain
- water breaks and not in labour after 6 hours
- feel ill
- swollen fingers, face and legs.

INFORMATION AND COUNSELLING SHEETS

PREPARING A BIRTH AND EMERGENCY PLAN

Preparing a birth plan

The health worker will provide you with information to help you prepare a birth plan. Based on your health condition, the health worker can make suggestions as to where it would be best to deliver. Whether in a hospital, health centre or at home, it is important to deliver with a skilled attendant.

AT EVERY VISIT TO THE HEALTH CENTRE, REVIEW AND DISCUSS YOUR BIRTH PLAN.
The plan can change if complications develop.

Planning for delivery at home

- Who do you choose to be the skilled attendant for delivery? How will you contact the skilled birth attendant to advise that you are in labour?
- Who will support you during labour and delivery?
- Who will be close by for at least 24 hours after delivery?
- Who will help you to care for your home and other children?
- Organize the following:
  → A clean and warm room or corner of a room.
  → Home-based maternal record.
  → A clean delivery kit which includes soap, a stick to clean under the nails, a new razor blade to cut the baby's cord, 3 pieces of string (about 20 cm. each) to tie the cord.
  → Clean cloths of different sizes: for the bed, for drying and wrapping the baby, for cleaning the baby's eyes, and for you to use as sanitary pads.
  → Warm covers for you and the baby.
  → Warm spot for the birth with a clean surface or clean cloth.
  → Bowls: two for washing and one for the placenta.
  → Plastic for wrapping the placenta.
  → Buckets of clean water and some way to heat this water.
  → For handwashing, water, soap and a towel or cloth for drying hands of the birth attendant.
  → Fresh drinking water, fluids and food for the mother.

Preparing an emergency plan

- To plan for an emergency, consider:
  → Where should you go?
  → How will you get there?
  → Will you have to pay for transport to get there? How much will it cost?
  → What costs will you have to pay at the health centre? How will you pay for this?
  → Can you start saving for these possible costs now?
  → Who will go with you to the health centre?
  → Who will help to care for your home and other children while you are away?

Planning for delivery at the hospital or health centre

- How will you get there? Will you have to pay for transport to get there?
- How much will it cost to deliver at the facility? How will you pay for this?
- Can you start saving for these costs now?
- Who will go with you and support you during labour and delivery?
- Who will help you while you are away and care for your home and other children?
- Bring the following:
  → Home-based maternal record.
  → Clean cloths of different sizes: for the bed, for drying and wrapping the baby, and for you to use as sanitary pads.
  → Clean clothes for you and the baby.
  → Food and water for you and the support person.

Care for the mother after birth

M4

CARE FOR THE MOTHER AFTER BIRTH

Care of the mother

- Eat more and healthier foods, including more meat, fish, oils, coconut, nuts, cereals, beans, vegetables, fruits, cheese and milk.
- Take iron tablets as explained by the health worker.
- Rest when you can.
- Drink plenty of clean, safe water.
- Sleep under a bednet treated with insecticide.
- Do not take medication unless prescribed at the health centre.
- Do not drink alcohol or smoke.
- Use a condom in every sexual relation, if you or your companion are at risk of sexually transmitted infections (STI) or HIV/AIDS.
- Wash all over daily, particularly the perineum.
- Change pad every 4 to 6 hours. Wash pad or dispose of it safely.

Family planning

- You can become pregnant within several weeks after delivery if you have sexual relations and are not breastfeeding exclusively.
- Talk to the health worker about choosing a family planning method which best meets your and your partner's needs.

Routine postnatal contacts

First contact: within 24 hours after childbirth

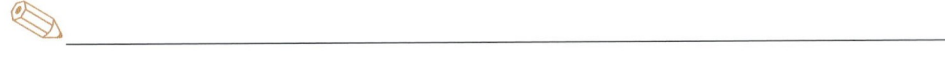

Second contact: on day 3 (48-72 hours)

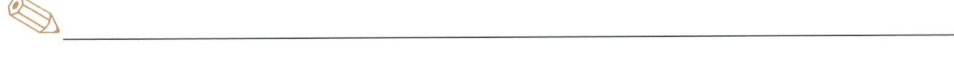

Third contact: between day 7 and 14 after birth.

Final postnatal contact (clinic visit): at 6 weeks after birth.

When to seek care for danger signs

Go to hospital or health centre **immediately, day or night, DO NOT** wait, if any of the following signs:
- Vaginal bleeding has increased.
- Fits.
- Fast or difficult breathing.
- Fever and too weak to get out of bed.
- Severe headaches with blurred vision.
- Calf pain, redness or swelling; shortness of breath or chest pain.

Go to health centre **as soon as possible** if any of the following signs:
- Swollen, red or tender breasts or nipples.
- Problems urinating, or leaking.
- Increased pain or infection in the perineum.
- Infection in the area of the wound.
- Smelly vaginal discharge.

CARE AFTER AN ABORTION

Self-care

- Some women prefer to rest for few days, especially if they feel tired
- It is normal for women to experience some vaginal bleeding (light, menstrual-like bleeding or spotting) for several weeks after an abortion.
- Some pain is normal after an abortion, as the uterus is contracting. A mild painkiller may help relieve cramping pain. If the pain increases over time, the woman should seek help.
- Do not have sexual intercourse or put anything into the vagina until bleeding stops.
- Practice safe sex and use a condom correctly in every act of sexual intercourse if at risk of STI or HIV.
- Return to the health worker as indicated.

Family planning

- Remember you can become pregnant as soon as you have sexual relations. Use a family planning method to prevent an unwanted pregnancy.
- Talk to the health worker about choosing a family planning method which best meets your and your partner's needs.

Know these danger signs

- If you have any of these signs, go to the health centre **immediately, day or night. DO NOT wait:**
- Increased bleeding.
- Fever, feeling ill.
- Dizziness or fainting.
- Abdominal pain.
- Backache.
- Nausea, vomiting.
- Foul-smelling vaginal discharge.

Additional support

- The health worker can help you identify persons or groups who can provide you with additional support if you should need it.

Care after an abortion M5

Care for the baby after birth — M6

CARE FOR THE BABY AFTER BIRTH

Care of the newborn

KEEP YOUR NEWBORN CLEAN

- Wash your baby's face and neck daily. Bathe her/him when necessary. After bathing, thoroughly dry your baby and then dress and keep her/him warm.
- Wash baby's bottom when soiled and dry it thoroughly.
- Wash your hands with soap and water before and after handling your baby, especially after touching her/his bottom.

CARE FOR THE NEWBORN'S UMBILICAL CORD

- Keep cord stump loosely covered with a clean cloth. Fold diaper and clothes below stump.
- Do not put anything on the stump. If the birth at home without a skilled attendant, apply 7.1% chlorhexidine digluconate (gel or liquid) to the stump daily for the first week of life.
- If stump area is soiled, wash with clean water and soap. Then dry completely with clean cloth.
- Wash your hands with soap and water before and after care.

KEEP YOUR NEWBORN WARM

- In cold climates, keep at least an area of the room warm.
- Newborns need more clothing than other children or adults.
- If cold, put a hat on the baby's head. During cold nights, cover the baby with an extra blanket.

OTHER ADVICE

- Let the baby sleep on her/his back or side.
- Keep the baby away from smoke.

Routine postnatal contacts

First contact: w<ithin 24 hours after childbirth.

_____

_____

Second contact: on day 3 (48-72 hours)

_____

_____

Third contact: between day 7 and 14 after birth.

_____

_____

Final postnatal contact (clinic visit): at 6 weeks after birth.
At these visits your baby will be vaccinated. **Have your baby immunized**.

When to seek care for danger signs

Go to hospital or health centre **immediately, day or night, DO NOT wait,** if your baby has any of the following signs:
- Difficulty breathing
- Fits
- Fever (temperature>=37.5 degrees celsius).
- Hypothermia<35.5 degrees celsius).
- Feels cold
- Bleeding
- Stops feeding
- Diarrhoea.

Go to the health centre **as soon as possible** if your baby has any of the following signs:
- Difficulty feeding.
- Feeds less than every 5 hours.
- Pus coming from the eyes.
- Irritated cord with pus or blood.
- Yellow eyes or skin.

BREASTFEEDING

Breastfeeding has many advantages

FOR THE BABY

- During the first 6 months of life, the baby needs nothing more than breast milk — not water, not other milk, not cereals, not teas, not juices.
- Breast milk contains exactly the water and nutrients that a baby's body needs. It is easily digested and efficiently used by the baby's body. It helps protect against infections and allergies and helps the baby's growth and development.

FOR THE MOTHER

- When the baby suckles, the uterus contracts. This helps reduce bleeding, but may be painful at first.
- Breastfeeding can help delay a new pregnancy.

FOR THE FIRST 6 MONTHS OF LIFE, GIVE ONLY BREAST MILK TO YOUR BABY, DAY AND NIGHT AS OFTEN AND AS LONG AS SHE/HE WANTS.

Suggestions for successful breastfeeding

- Immediately after birth, keep your baby in the bed with you, or within easy reach.
- Start breastfeeding within 1 hour of birth.
- The baby's suckling stimulates your milk production. The more the baby feeds, the more milk you will produce.
- At each feeding, let the baby feed and release your breast, and then offer your second breast. At the next feeding, alternate and begin with the second breast.
- Give your baby the first milk (colostrum). It is nutritious and has antibodies to help keep your baby healthy.
- At night, let your baby sleep with you, within easy reach.
- While breastfeeding, you should drink plenty of clean, safe water. You should eat more and healthier foods and rest when you can.

The health worker can support you in starting and maintaining breastfeeding

- The health worker can help you to correctly position the baby and ensure she/he attaches to the breast. This will reduce breast problems for the mother.
- The health worker can show you how to express milk from your breast with your hands. If you should need to leave the baby with another caretaker for short periods, you can leave your milk and it can be given to the baby in a cup.
- The health worker can put you in contact with a breastfeeding support group.

If you have any difficulties with breastfeeding, see the health worker immediately.

Breastfeeding and family planning

- During the first 6 months after birth, if you breastfeed exclusively, day and night, and your menstruation has not returned, you are protected against another pregnancy.
- If you do not meet these requirements, or if you wish to use another family planning method while breastfeeding, discuss the different options available with the health worker.

Clean home delivery (1) M8

CLEAN HOME DELIVERY

Regardless of the site of delivery, it is strongly recommended that all women deliver with a skilled attendant.
For a woman who prefers to deliver at home the following recommendations are provided for a clean home delivery to be reviewed during antenatal care visits.

Delivery at home with an attendant

- Ensure the attendant and other family members know the emergency plan and are aware of danger signs for yourself and your baby.
- Arrange for a support person to assist the attendant and to stay with you during labour and after delivery.
  - Have these supplies organized for a clean delivery: new razor blade, 3 pieces of string about 20 cm each to tie the cord, 7.1% chlorhexidine digluconate (gel or liquid) for umbilical cord care [where recommended by health authority] and clean cloths to cover the birth place.
  - Prepare the home and the supplies indicated for a safe birth:
    - Clean, warm birth place with fresh air and a source of light
    - Clean warm blanket to cover you
  - Clean cloths:
    - for drying and wrapping the baby
    - for cleaning the baby's eyes
    - to use as sanitary pads after birth
    - to dry your body after washing
    - for birth attendant to dry her hands.
  - Clean clothes for you to wear after delivery
  - Fresh drinking water, fluids and food for you
  - Buckets of clean water and soap for washing, for you and the skilled attendant
  - Means to heat water
  - Three bowls, two for washing and one for the placenta
  - Plastic for wrapping the placenta
  - Bucket for you to urinate in.

Instructions to woman and family for a clean and safer delivery at home

- Make sure there is a clean delivery surface for the birth of the baby.
- Ask the attendant to wash her hands before touching you or the baby. The nails of the attendant should be short and clean.
- When the baby is born, place her/him on your abdomen/chest where it is warm and clean. Dry the baby thoroughly and wipe the face with a clean cloth. Then cover with a clean dry cloth.
- Cut the cord when it stops pulsating, using the disposable delivery kit, according to instructions.
- Wait for the placenta to deliver on its own.
- Make sure you and your baby are warm. Have the baby near you, dressed or wrapped and with head covered with a cap.
- Start breastfeeding when the baby shows signs of readiness, within the first hour of birth.
- Where recommended by the health authority, apply 7.1% chlorhexidine digluconate (gel or liquid) to the umbilical cord stump daily for the first week of life. Where chlorhexidine is not used for umbilical cord care, keep cord clean and dry.
- Dispose of placenta (using safe and culturally accepted way to dispose placenta).

- **DO NOT** be alone for the 24 hours after delivery.
- **DO NOT** bath the baby on the first day.

Avoid harmful practices

FOR EXAMPLE:
Do not use local medications to hasten labour.
Do not wait for waters to stop before going to health facility.
Do not insert any substances into the vagina during labour or after delivery.
Do not push on the abdomen during labour or delivery.
Do not pull on the cord to deliver the placenta.
Do not put any substance on umbilical cord/stump other than 7.1% chlorhexidine digluconate (where recommended by health authority).

_____

_____

Encourage helpful traditional practices:

_____

_____

Danger signs during delivery

If you or your baby has any of these signs, **go to the hospital or health centre immediately, day or night, Do not wait.**

MOTHER
- If waters break and not in labour after 6 hours.
- Labour pains (contractions) continue for more than 12 hours.
- Heavy bleeding (soaks more than 2-3 pads in 15 minutes).
- Placenta not expelled 1 hour after birth of baby.

BABY
- Very small.
- Difficulty in breathing.
- Fits.
- Fever.
- Feels cold.
- Bleeding.
- Not able to feed.

Routine postnatal contacts

- If birth is at home, the first postnatal contact should be as early as possible within 24 hours of birth.
- Second contact: on day 3 (48-72 hours).
- Third contact: between day 7 and 14 after birth.
- Final postnatal contact (clinic visit): at 6 weeks after birth.

Clean home delivery (2)

M9

RECORDS AND FORMS

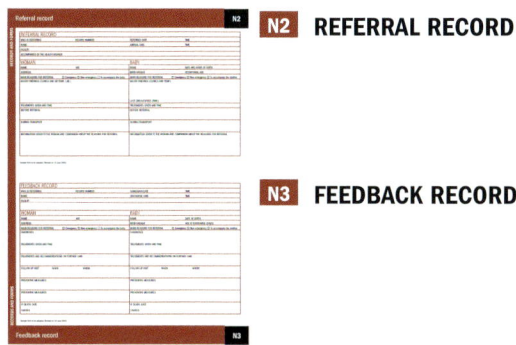

N2 REFERRAL RECORD

N3 FEEDBACK RECORD

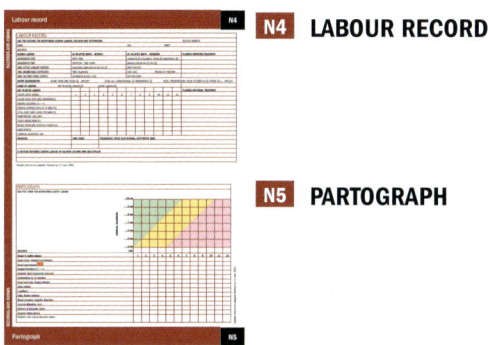

N4 LABOUR RECORD

N5 PARTOGRAPH

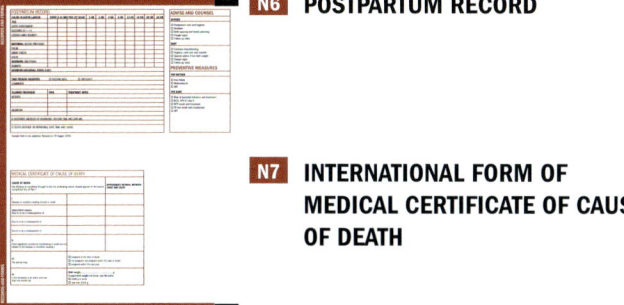

N6 POSTPARTUM RECORD

N7 INTERNATIONAL FORM OF MEDICAL CERTIFICATE OF CAUSE OF DEATH

- Records are suggested not so much for the format as for the content.
  The content of the records is adjusted to the content of the Guide.

- Modify national or local records to include all the relevant sections needed to record important information for the provider, the woman and her family, for the purposes of monitoring and surveillance and official reporting.

- Fill out other required records such as immunization cards for the mother and baby.

Referral record

N2

REFERRAL RECORD

WHO IS REFERRING	RECORD NUMBER	REFERRED DATE	TIME
NAME		ARRIVAL DATE	TIME
FACILITY			
ACCOMPANIED BY THE HEALTH WORKER			

WOMAN | BAQY

WOMAN		BABY	
NAME	AGE	NAME	DATE AND HOUR OF BIRTH
ADDRESS		BIRTH WEIGHT	GESTATIONAL AGE
MAIN REASONS FOR REFERRAL ☐ Emergency ☐ Non-emergency ☐ To accompany the baby		MAIN REASONS FOR REFERRAL ☐ Emergency ☐ Non-emergency ☐ To accompany the mother	
MAJOR FINDINGS (CLINICA AND BP, TEMP., LAB.)		MAJOR FINDINGS (CLINICA AND TEMP.)	
		LAST (BREAST)FEED (TIME)	
TREATMENTS GIVEN AND TIME		TREATMENTS GIVEN AND TIME	
BEFORE REFERRAL		BEFORE REFERRAL	
DURING TRANSPORT		DURING TRANSPORT	
INFORMATION GIVEN TO THE WOMAN AND COMPANION ABOUT THE REASONS FOR REFERRAL		INFORMATION GIVEN TO THE WOMAN AND COMPANION ABOUT THE REASONS FOR REFERRAL	

Sample form to be adapted.

FEEDBACK RECORD

WHO IS REFERRING	RECORD NUMBER	ADMISSION DATE	TIME
NAME		DISCHARGE DATE	TIME
FACILITY			

WOMAN

NAME	AGE
ADDRESS	
MAIN REASONS FOR REFERRAL	☐ Emergency ☐ Non-emergency ☐ To accompany the baby
DIAGNOSES	
TREATMENTS GIVEN AND TIME	
TREATMENTS AND RECOMMENDATIONS ON FURTHER CARE	
FOLLOW-UP VISIT	WHEN	WHERE
PREVENTIVE MEASURES	
PREVENTIVE MEASURES	
IF DEATH: DATE	
CAUSES	

BABY

NAME	DATE OF BIRTH
BIRTH WEIGHT	AGE AT DISCHARGE (DAYS)
MAIN REASONS FOR REFERRAL	☐ Emergency ☐ Non-emergency ☐ To accompany the mother
DIAGNOSES	
TREATMENTS GIVEN AND TIME	
TREATMENTS AND RECOMMENDATIONS ON FURTHER CARE	
FOLLOW-UP VISIT	WHEN	WHERE
PREVENTIVE MEASURES	
PREVENTIVE MEASURES	
IF DEATH: DATE	
CAUSES	

Sample form to be adapted.

Feedback record

Labour record

N4

LABOUR RECORD

USE THIS RECORD FOR MONITORING DURING LABOUR, DELIVERY AND POSTPARTUM

RECORD NUMBER

NAME		AGE	PARITY	
ADDRESS				
DURING LABOUR	**AT OR AFTER BIRTH – MOTHER**	**AT OR AFTER BIRTH – NEWBORN**		**PLANNED NEWBORN TREATMENT**
ADMISSION DATE	BIRTH TIME	LIVEBIRTH ☐ STILLBIRTH: FRESH ☐ MACERATED ☐		
ADMISSION TIME	OXYTOCIN – TIME GIVEN	RESUSCITATION NO ☐ YES ☐		
TIME ACTIVE LABOUR STARTED	PLACENTA COMPLETE NO ☐ YES ☐	BIRTH WEIGHT		
TIME MEMBRANES RUPTURED	TIME DELIVERED	GEST. AGE	WEEKS OR PRETERM	
TIME SECOND STAGE STARTS	ESTIMATED BLOOD LOSS	SECOND BABY		

ENTRY EXAMINATION   MORE THAN ONE FETUS ☐ - SPECIFY   FETAL LIE: LONGITUDINAL ☐ TRANSVERSE ☐   FETAL PRESENTATION: HEAD ☐ BREECH ☐ OTHER ☐ - SPECIFY

STAGE OF LABOUR   NOT IN ACTIVE LABOUR ☐   ACTIVE LABOUR ☐

NOT IN ACTIVE LABOUR													**PLANNED MATERNAL TREATMENT**
HOURS SINCE ARRIVAL	1	2	3	4	5	6	7	8	9	10	11	12	
HOURS SINCE RUPTURED MEMBRANES													
VAGINAL BLEEDING (0 + ++)													
STRONG CONTRACTIONS IN 10 MINUTES													
FETAL HEART RATE (BEATS PER MINUTE)													
TEMPERATURE (AXILLARY)													
PULSE (BEATS/MINUTE)													
BLOOD PRESSURE (SYSTOLIC/DIASTOLIC)													
URINE VOIDED													
CERVICAL DILATATION (CM)													

PROBLEM	**TIME ONSET**	**TREATMENTS OTHER THAN NORMAL SUPPORTIVE CARE**

IF MOTHER REFERRED DURING LABOUR OR DELIVERY, RECORD TIME AND EXPLAIN

Sample form to be adapted.

PARTOGRAPH

USE THIS FORM FOR MONITORING ACTIVE LABOUR

CERVICAL DILATATION

10 cm
9 cm
8 cm
7 cm
6 cm
5 cm
4 cm

TIME

FINDINGS												
Hours in active labour	1	2	3	4	5	6	7	8	9	10	11	12
Hours since ruptured membranes												
Rapid assessment B3-B7												
Vaginal bleeding (0 + ++)												
Amniotic fluid (meconium stained)												
Contractions in 10 minutes												
Fetal heart rate (beats/minute)												
Urine voided												
T (axillary)												
Pulse (beats/minute)												
Blood pressure (systolic/diastolic)												
Cervical dilatation (cm)												
Delivery of placenta (time)												
Oxytocin (time/given)												
Problem-note onset/describe below												

Sample form to be adapted. Revised on 13 June 2003.

RECORDS AND FORMS

Partograph

Postpartum record

N6

POSTPARTUM RECORD

HOURS IN ACTIVE LABOUR	EVERY 5-15 MIN FOR 1ST HOUR	2 HR	3 HR	4 HR	8 HR	12 HR	16 HR	20 HR	24 HR
TIME									
RAPID ASSESSMENT									
BLEEDING (0 + ++)									
UTERUS HARD/ROUND?									
MATERNAL: BLOOD PRESSURE									
PULSE									
URINE VOIDED									
VULVA									
NEWBORN: BREATHING									
WARMTH									
NEWBORN ABNORMAL SIGNS (LIST)									

TIME FEEDING OBSERVED	☐ FEEDING WELL	☐ DIFFICULTY
COMMENTS		

PLANNED TREATMENT	TIME	TREATMENT GIVEN
MOTHER		
NEWBORN		

IF REFERRED (MOTHER OR NEWBORN), RECORD TIME AND EXPLAIN:

IF DEATH (MOTHER OR NEWBORN), DATE, TIME AND CAUSE:

Sample form to be adapted.

ADVISE AND COUNSEL

MOTHER

☐ Postpartum care and hygiene
☐ Nutrition
☐ Birth spacing and family planning
☐ Danger signs
☐ Follow-up visits

BABY

☐ Exclusive breastfeeding
☐ Hygiene, cord care and warmth
☐ Special advice if low birth weight
☐ Danger signs
☐ Follow-up visits

PREVENTIVE MEASURES

FOR MOTHER

☐ Iron/folate
☐ Mebendazole
☐ ART

FOR BABY

☐ Risk of bacterial infection and treatment
☐ BCG, OPV-0, Hep-0
☐ RPR result and treatment
☐ TB test result and prophylaxis
☐ ART

MEDICAL CERTIFICATE OF CAUSE OF DEATH

CAUSE OF DEATH *the disease or condition thought to be the underlying cause should appear in the lowest completed line of Part I*		**APPROXIMATE INTERVAL BETWEEN ONSET AND DEATH**
I Disease or condition leading directly to death		
Antecedent causes: Due to or as a consequence of		
Due to or as a consequence of		
Due to or as a consequence of		
II Other significant conditions Contributing to death but not related to the disease or condition causing it		
III The woman was:	☐ pregnant at the time of death ☐ not pregnant, but pregnant within 42 days of death ☐ pregnant within the past year	
IV If the deceased is an infant and less than one month old	Birth weight:................................g If exact birth weight not know, was the baby: ☐ 2500 g or more ☐ less than 2500 g	

International form of medical certificate of cause of death

N7

Glossary

GLOSSARY

ABORTION

Termination of pregnancy from whatever cause before the fetus is capable of extrauterine life.

ADOLESCENT

Young person 10–19 years old.

ADVISE

To give information and suggest to someone a course of action.

ANTENATAL CARE

Care for the woman and fetus during pregnancy.

ASSESS

To consider the relevant information and make a judgement. As used in this guide, to examine a woman or baby and identify signs of illness.

BABY

A very young boy or girl in the first week(s) of life.

BIRTH

Expulsion or extraction of the baby (regardless of whether the cord has been cut).

BIRTH AND EMERGENCY PLAN

A plan for safe childbirth developed in antenatal care visit which considers the woman's condition, preferences and available resources. A plan to seek care for danger signs during pregnancy, childbirth and postpartum period, for the woman and newborn.

BIRTH WEIGHT

The first of the fetus or newborn obtained after birth.

For live births, birth weight should preferably be measured within the first hour of life before significant postnatal weight loss has occurred, recorded to the degree of accuracy to which it is measured.

CHART

As used in this guide, a sheet presenting information in the form of a table.

CHILDBIRTH

Giving birth to a baby or babies and placenta.

CLASSIFY

To select a category of illness and severity based on a woman's or baby's signs and symptoms.

CLINIC

As used in this guide, any first-level outpatient health facility such as a dispensary, rural health post, health centre or outpatient department of a hospital.

COMMUNITY

As used in this guide, a group of people sometimes living in a defined geographical area, who share common culture, values and norms. Economic and social differences need to be taken into account when determining needs and establishing links within a given community.

BIRTH COMPANION

Partner, other family member or friend who accompanies the woman during labour and delivery.

CHILDBEARING AGE (WOMAN)

15-49 years. As used in this guide, also a girl 10-14 years, or a woman more than 49 years, when pregnant, after abortion, after delivery.

COMPLAINT

As described in this guide, the concerns or symptoms of illness or complication need to be assessed and classified in order to select treatment.

CONCERN

A worry or an anxiety that the woman may have about herself or the baby(ies).

COMPLICATION

A condition occurring during pregnancy or aggravating it. This classification includes conditions such as obstructed labour or bleeding.

CONFIDENCE

A feeling of being able to succeed.

CONTRAINDICATION

A condition occurring during another disease or aggravating it. This classification includes conditions such as obstructed labour or bleeding.

COUNSELLING

As used in this guide, interaction with a woman to support her in solving actual or anticipated problems, reviewing options, and making decisions. It places emphasis on provider support for helping the woman make decisions.

DANGER SIGNS

Terminology used to explain to the woman the signs of life-threatening and other serious conditions which require immediate intervention.

EMERGENCY SIGNS

Signs of life-threatening conditions which require immediate intervention.

ESSENTIAL

Basic, indispensable, necessary.

FACILITY

A place where organized care is provided: a health post, health centre, hospital maternity or emergency unit, or ward.

FAMILY

Includes relationships based on blood, marriage, sexual partnership, and adoption, and a broad range of groups whose bonds are based on feelings of trust mutual support, and a shared destiny.

Glossary

FOLLOW-UP VISIT
A return visit requested by a health worker to see if further treatment or referral is needed.

GESTATIONAL AGE
Duration of pregnancy from the last menstrual period. In this guide, duration of pregnancy (gestational age) is expressed in 3 different ways:

Trimester	Months	Weeks
First	less than 4 months	less than 16 weeks
Second	4-6 months	16-28 weeks
Third	7-9+ months	29-40+ weeks

GRUNTING
Soft short sounds that a baby makes when breathing out. Grunting occurs when a baby is having difficulty breathing.

HOME DELIVERY
Delivery at home (with a skilled attendant, a traditional birth attendant, a family member, or by the woman herself).

HOSPITAL
As used in this guide, any health facility with inpatient beds, supplies and expertise to treat a woman or newborn with complications.

INTEGRATED MANAGEMENT
A process of caring for the woman in pregnancy, during and after childbirth, and for her newborn, that includes considering all necessary elements: care to ensure they remain healthy, and prevention, detection and management of complications in the context of her environment and according to her wishes.

LABOUR
As used in this guide, a period from the onset of regular contractions to complete delivery of the placenta.

LOW BIRTH WEIGHT BABY
Weighing less than 2500-g at birth.

MATERNITY CLINIC
Health centre with beds or a hospital where women and their newborns receive care during childbirth and delivery, and emergency first aid.

MISCARRIAGE
Or spontaneous abortion. Premature expulsion of a non-viable fetus from the uterus.

MONITORING
Frequently repeated measurements of vital signs or observations of danger signs.

NEWBORN
Recently born infant. In this guide used interchangeable with baby.

PARTNER
As used in this guide, the male companion of the pregnant woman (husband, "free union") who is the father of the baby or the actual sexual partner.

POSTNATAL CARE
Care for the baby after birth. For the purposes of this guide, up to two weeks.

POSTPARTUM CARE
Care for the woman provided in the postpartum period, e.g. from complete delivery of the placenta to 42 days after delivery.

PRE-REFERRAL
Before referral to a hospital.

PREGNANCY
Period from when the woman misses her menstrual period or the uterus can be felt, to the onset of labour/elective caesarian section or abortion.

PREMATURE
Before 37 completed weeks of pregnancy.

PRETERM BABY
Born early, before 37 completed weeks of pregnancy. If number of weeks not known, 1 month early.

PRIMARY HEALTH CARE*
Essential health care accessible at a cost the country and community can afford, with methods that are practical, scientifically sound and socially acceptable. (Among the essential activities are maternal and child health care, including family planning; immunization; appropriate treatment of common diseases and injuries; and the provision of essential drugs).

PRIMARY HEALTH CARE LEVEL
Health post, health centre or maternity clinic; a hospital providing care for normal pregnancy and childbirth.

PRIORITY SIGNS
Signs of serious conditions which require interventions as soon as possible, before they become life-threatening.

QUICK CHECK
A quick check assessment of the health status of the woman or her baby at the first contact with the health provider or services in order to assess if emergency care is required.

RAPID ASSESSMENT AND MANAGEMENT
Systematic assessment of vital functions of the woman and the most severe presenting signs and symptoms; immediate initial management of the life-threatening conditions; and urgent and safe referral to the next level of care.

REASSESSMENT
As used in this guide, to examine the woman or baby again for signs of a specific illness or condition to see if she or the newborn are improving.

RECOMMENDATION
Advice. Instruction that should be followed.

REFERRAL, URGENT
As used in this guide, sending a woman or baby, or both, for further assessment and care to a higher level of care; including arranging for transport and care during transport, preparing written information (referral form), and communicating with the referral institution.

REFERRAL HOSPITAL
A hospital with a full range of obstetric services including surgery and blood transfusion and care for newborns with problems.

Glossary

REINFECTION

Infection with same or a different strain of HIV virus.

REPLACEMENT FEEDING

The process of feeding a baby who is not receiving breast milk with a diet that provides all the nutrients she/he needs until able to feed entirely on family foods.

SECONDARY HEALTH CARE

More specialized care offered at the most peripheral level, for example radiographic diagnostic, general surgery, care of women with complications of pregnancy and childbirth, and diagnosis and treatment of uncommon and severe diseases. (This kind of care is provided by trained staff at such institutions as district or provincial hospitals).

SHOCK

A dangerous condition with severe weakness, lethargy, or unconsciousness, cold extremeties, and fast, weak pulse. It is caused by severe bleeding, severe infection, or obstructed labour.

SIGN

As used in this guide, physical evidence of a health problem which the health worker observes by looking, listening, feeling or measuring. Examples of signs: bleeding, convulsions, hypertension, anaemia, fast breathing.

SKILLED ATTENDANT

Refers exclusively to people with midwifery skills (for example, midwives, doctors and nurses) who have been trained to proficiency in the skills necessary to manage normal deliveries and diagnose or refer obstetric complications.

For the purposes of this guide, a person with midwifery skills who:

- has acquired the requisite qualifications to be registered and/or legally licensed to practice training and licensing requirements are country-specific;
- May practice in hospitals, clinics, health units, in the home, or in any other service setting.
- Is able to do the following:
  → give necessary care and advice to women during pregnancy and postpartum and for their newborn infants;
  → conduct deliveries on her/his own and care for the mother and newborn; this includes provision of preventive care, and detection and appropriate referral of abnormal conditions.
  → provide emergency care for the woman and newborn; perform selected obstetrical procedures such as manual removal of placenta and newborn resuscitation; prescribe and give drugs (IM/IV) and infusions to the mother and baby as needed, including for post-abortion care.
  → provide health information and counselling for the woman, her family and community.

SMALL BABY

A newly born infant born preterm and/or with low birth weight.

STABLE

Staying the same rather than getting worse.

STILLBIRTH

Birth of a baby that shows no signs of life at birth (no gasping, breathing or heart beat).

SURVEILLANCE, PERMANENT

Continuous presence and observation of a woman in labour.

SYMPTOM

As used in this guide, a health problem reported by a woman, such as pain or headache.

TERM, FULL-TERM

Word used to describe a baby born after 37 completed weeks of pregnancy.

TRIMESTER OF PREGNANCY

See Gestational age.

VERY SMALL BABY

Baby with birth weight less than 1500 g or gestational age less than 32 weeks.

WHO definitions have been used where possible but, for the purposes of this guide, have been modified where necessary to be more appropriate to clinical care (reasons for modification are given). For conditions where there are no official WHO definitions, operational terms are proposed, again only for the purposes of this guide.

ACRONYMS

AIDS Acquired immunodeficiency syndrome, caused by infection with human immunodeficiency virus (HIV). AIDS is the final and most severe phase of HIV infection.

ANC Care for the woman and fetus during pregnancy.

ART The use of a combination of three or more antiretroviral drugs for treating a pregnant and breastfeeding woman with HIV infection for their own health and to prevent the transmission of HIV to her baby.

ARV Antiretroviral drugs refer to the medicines themselves and not their use.

BCG An immunization to prevent tuberculosis, given at birth.

BP Blood pressure.

BPM Beats per minute.

FHR Fetal heart rate.

Hb Haemoglobin.

HB-1 Vaccine given at birth to prevent hepatitis B.

HMBR Home-based maternal record: pregnancy, delivery and inter-pregnancy record for the woman and some information about the newborn.

HIV Human immunodeficiency virus. HIV is the virus that causes AIDS.

INH Isoniazid, a drug to treat tuberculosis.

IV Intravenous (injection or infusion).

IM Intramuscular injection.

IU International unit.

IUD Intrauterine device.

LAM Lactation amenorrhea.

LBW Low birth weight: birth weight less than 2500 g.

LMP Last menstrual period: a date from which the date of delivery is estimated.

MTCT Mother-to-child transmission of HIV.

NG Naso-gastric tube, a feeding tube put into the stomach through the nose.

ORS Oral rehydration solution.

OPV-0 Oral polio vaccine. To prevent poliomyelitis, OPV-0 is given at birth.

QC A quick check assessment of the health status of the woman or her baby at the first contact with the health provider or services in order to assess if emergency care is required.

RAM Systematic assessment of vital functions of the woman and the most severe presenting signs and symptoms; immediate initial management of the life-threatening conditions; and urgent and safe referral to the next level of care.

RPR Rapid plasma reagin, a rapid test for syphilis. It can be performed in the clinic.

STI Sexually transmitted infection.

TT An immunization against tetanus

> More than

≥ Equal or more than

< Less than

≤ Equal or less than